WHO Technical Report Series
923

RHEUMATIC FEVER AND RHEUMATIC HEART DISEASE

Report of a WHO Expert Consultation
Geneva, 29 October – 1 November 2001

GW00728793

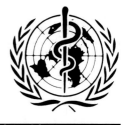

World Health Organization
Geneva 2004

WHO Library Cataloguing-in-Publication Data

WHO Expert Consultation on Rheumatic Fever and Rheumatic Heart Disease
(2001 : Geneva, Switzerland)
Rheumatic fever and rheumatic heart disease : report of a WHO Expert Consultation,
Geneva, 29 October — 1 November 2001.

(WHO technical report series ; 923)

1.Rheumatic fever 2.Rheumatic heart disease 3.Endocarditis 4.Cost of illness I.Title
II.Series

ISBN 92 4 120923 2   (NLM classification: WC 220)
ISSN 0512-3054

Typeset in Hong Kong
Printed in Singapore
2003/15621

Contents

WHO Expert Consultation on Rheumatic Fever and Rheumatic Heart Disease

Geneva, 29 October–1 November 2001

Members

Alan Bisno, Department of Medicine, Veterans Administration Medical Center, Miami, Florida, USA.

Eric G Butchart, Director, Cardiothoracic Surgery, University Hospital, Cardiff, Wales, UK.

NK Ganguly, Director-General, Indian Council of Medical Research, New Delhi, India.

Tesfamicael Ghebrehiwet, Consultant, Nursing & Health Policy, International Council of Nurses, Geneva, Switzerland.

Hung-Chi Lue, Professor of Pediatrics, National Taiwan University Hospital, Taipei, Taiwan.

Edward L Kaplan, Department of Pediatrics, University of Minnesota Medical School, Minneapolis, MN, USA. (**Co-Chair**).

Nawal Kordofani, Programme Coordinator, RF/RHD Prevention Programme, Shaab Teaching Hospital, Khartoum, Sudan.

Diana Martin, Principal Scientist, Institute of Environmental Science & Research, Kenepuro Science Centre, Porirua, New Zealand.

Doreen Millard, Consultant Paediatrician, Paediatrics & Paediatric Cardiology, Kingston, Jamaica.

Jagat Narula, Hahnemann University School of Medicine, Philadelphia, USA. (**Co-Rapporteur**).

Diego Vanuzzo, Servizio di Prevenzione Cardiovascolari, Centro per la Lotta alle Malattie Cardiovascolari, P. le Santa Maria Misericordia, Udine, Italy.

Salah RA Zaher, Assistant Professor of Pediatrics, University of Alexandria, Alexandria, Egypt. (**Co-Rapporteur**).

WHO Secretariat

Derek Yach, Executive Director, Noncommunicable and Mental Health Cluster (NMH).

Rafael Bengoa, Director, Management of Noncommunicable Diseases (MNC).

Shanthi Mendis, Coordinator, Cardiovascular Disease (CVD). (**Co-Chair**).

Porfirio Nordet, Cardiovascular Disease (CVD).

Dele Abegunde, Cardiovascular Disease (CVD).

Francesca Celletti, Cardiovascular Disease (CVD).

Claus Heuck, Blood Safety and Clinical Technology, Diagnostic Imaging and Laboratory Technology (BCT/DIL).

1. Introduction

A WHO Expert Consultation on Rheumatic Fever (RF) and Rheumatic Heart Disease (RHD) met in WHO/HQ, Geneva from 29 October to 1 November 2001 to update the WHO Technical Report 764 on Rheumatic Fever and Rheumatic Heart Disease, first published in 1988 (*1*). Dr. Rafael Bengoa, Director Division of Management Noncommunicable Diseases, opened the meeting on behalf of the Director-General.

RF and RHD remain significant causes of cardiovascular diseases in the world today. Despite a documented decrease in the incidence of acute RF and a similar documented decrease in the prevalence of RHD in industrialized countries during the past five decades, these non-suppurative cardiovascular sequel of group A streptococcal pharyngitis remain medical and public health problems in *both* industrialized and industrializing countries even at the beginning of the 21st century. The most devastating effects are on children and young adults in their most productive years.

For at least five decades this unique non-suppurative sequel to group A streptococcal infections has been a concern of the World Health Organization and its member countries. Sentinel studies conducted under the auspices of the WHO during the last four decades clearly documented that the control of the preceding infections and their sequelae is both cost effective and inexpensive. Without doubt, appropriate public health control programs and optimal medical care reduce the burden of disease (1–6).

Although the responsible pathogenic mechanism(s) still remain incompletely defined, methods for optimal prevention and management have changed during the past fifteen years (5–8). To make this information available to physicians and public health authorities, WHO convened this expert consultation to both update and to expand the 1988 document. RF and RHD remain to be conquered, but until that can be accomplished, optimal methods of prevention and management are required. The recommendations in this document are based upon current medical literature. Every attempt has been made to make this a practically useful document and at the same time to furnish appropriate references with additional information for the practitioner.

References

1. *Rheumatic fever and rheumatic heart disease. Report of a WHO Study Group.* World Health Organization, Geneva, 1988 (Technical Report Series No. 764).

2. *Prevention of rheumatic fever. Report of a WHO Expert Committee.* World Health Organization, Geneva, 1966 (Technical Report Series No. 342).

3. **Strasser T et al.** The community control of rheumatic fever and rheumatic heart disease: report of a WHO international cooperative project. *Bulletin of the World Health Organization,* 1981, **59**(2):285–294.

4. WHO/CVD unit and principal investigators. WHO programme for the prevention of rheumatic fever/rheumatic heart disease in sixteen developing countries: report from Phase I (1986–1990). *Bulletin of the World Health Organization,* 1992, **70**(2):213–218.

5. *Joint WHO/ISFC meeting on rheumatic fever/rheumatic heart disease control with emphasis on primary prevention, Geneva, 7–9 September 1994.* Geneva, World Health Organization, 1994 (WHO/CVD 94.1).

6. *The WHO global programme for the prevention of RF/RHD. Report of a consultation to review progress and develop future activities.* Geneva, World Health Organization, 2000 (WHO/CVD/00.1).

7. **Narula J et al.** *Rheumatic fever.* Washington, DC, American Registry of Pathology Publisher, 1999.

8. **Stevens D, Kaplan E.** *Streptococcal infections. Clinical aspects, microbiology, and molecular pathogenesis.* New York, Oxford University Press, 2000.

2. Epidemiology of group A streptococci, rheumatic fever and rheumatic heart disease

Rheumatic fever (RF) and rheumatic heart disease (RHD) are nonsuppurative complications of Group A streptococcal pharyngitis due to a delayed immune response. Although RF and RHD are rare in developed countries, they are still major public health problems among children and young adults in developing countries (1–6). The economic effects of the disability and premature death caused by these diseases are felt at both the individual and national levels through higher direct and indirect health-care costs.

Group A streptococcal infections

Beta-haemolytic streptococci can be divided into a number of serological groups on the basis of their cell-wall polysaccharide antigen. Those in serological group A (*Streptococcus pyogenes*) can be further subdivided into more than 130 distinct M types, and are responsible for the vast majority of infections in humans (7–9). Furthermore, only pharyngitis caused by group A streptococci has been linked with the etiopathogenesis of RF and RHD. Other streptococcal groups (e.g. B, C, G and F) have been isolated from human subjects and are sometimes associated with infection; and streptococci in groups C and G can produce extracellular antigens (including streptolysin-O) with similar characteristics to that produced by group A streptococci (7–9). Nevertheless, the available evidence does not link streptococci in non-group A types with the pathogenesis of RF and RHD, although further studies are warranted into the role of groups C and G in the pathogenesis of RF (1, 2, 7–9).

In both developing and developed countries, pharyngitis and skin infection (impetigo) are the most common infections caused by group A streptococci. Group A streptococci are the most common bacterial cause of pharyngitis, with a peak incidence in children 5–15 years of age (3, 5, 7, 9). Streptococcal pharyngitis is less frequent among children in the first three years of life and among adults. It has been estimated that most children develop at least one episode of pharyngitis per year, 15–20% of which are caused by group A streptococci and nearly 80% by viral pathogens (1, 5, 7, 9). The incidence of pharyngeal beta-haemolytic streptococcal infections can vary between countries and within the same country, depending upon season, age group, socioeconomic conditions, environmental factors and the quality of health care (1–3, 5, 10, 11). Surveys of healthy schoolchildren 6–10 years of age, for example, found anti-streptolysin-O titres >200 Todd units in 15–70% of the children (2), while other studies reported beta-haemolytic streptococci carrier rates of 10–50% for asymptomatic schoolchildren (*1, 2*). In temperate countries, 50–60% of streptococci isolated from asymptomatic children belong to serological group A, while streptococci in serological groups C and G together occur in less than 30% of the children. Conversely, in many tropical countries, groups C and G streptococci occur with rates as high as 60–70% in asymptomatic carriers (*1–3, 5, 11*).

The presence of group A streptococci in the upper respiratory tract (URT) may reflect either true infection or a carrier state. In either state, the patient harbours the organism, but only in the case of a true infection does the patient show a rising antibody response. In the carrier state there is no rising antibody response. It is thought that a patient with a true infection is at risk of developing RF and of spreading the organism to close contacts, while this is not thought to be the case with carriers (*1, 5, 10*). Therefore, many professionals feel that only patients with true infections need to be given antibiotics. (For alternative characterizations of the streptococcal carrier state see reference *10*).

Under endemic conditions, group A streptococci have been isolated from patients with symptomatic pharyngitis. Recovery rates varied from 13.5% in Northern India, to 33% in Utrecht, Netherlands, and to 44% in Zagreb, Croatia (Table 2.1; *12–18*). Group A streptococci are highly transmissible and spread rapidly in families and communities, with the predominant M types constantly changing. However, in publications about RF outbreaks, including recent ones in the United

Table 2.1
Examples of presence of group A beta-haemolytic streptococci in children with symptomatic pharyngitis

Source	Year	City/country	Patients with pharyngitis (N)	GAβHS positive (%)[a]
14	1980s	Rhode Island, USA	8668 (5–19 years old)	24.3
15	1987	Havana, Cuba	480	25.0
				34.5[b]
12	1995	Northern India	910	13.5
16	1993	Cairo, Egypt	451	24.0
17	1997	Utrecht, Netherlands	558	33.0
				75.0[b]
18	1992	Creteil, France	307	36.8
13	1992	Zagreb, Croatia	629	44.7

[a] GAβHS positive = patients positive for group A beta-haemolytic streptococci.
[b] Patients with clinical features of streptococcal pharyngitis (fever > 38 °C; tonsilar exudate, anterior cervical lymphadenopathiy and absence of cough, rhinorrhea and conjunctivitis.

States of America (USA), it was reported that only a limited number of streptococcal stereotypes (i.e. M serotypes 1, 3, 5, 6, 18, 19, 24) were obtained from the throat cultures of children in the affected communities (*2, 3, 5, 7, 19–23*).

Although no longitudinal studies have examined trends in group A streptococcal pharyngitis, nor in the asymptomatic carrier rates, available data suggest that pharyngitis and asymptomatic carrier rates have remained more-or-less stable in most countries (*3, 5*). However, in the last 20 years, some countries have reported changes in the M types, severity and other characteristics of group A streptococci. More-virulent strains have re-emerged, for example, and non-M type streptococci have been detected (*1–3, 5, 7, 11, 22*). In the USA, despite a remarkable reduction in the incidence of RF since the 1950s, the incidence of URT infections caused by group A streptococci has not declined (*1–3, 5, 20, 23*). In the mid-1980s, the virulence, severity and sequelae of these infections also appear to have changed remarkably. Outbreaks of acute RF have been described from widely separated areas of the country, and complications of streptococcal infections have been reported, including necrotising fascitis, streptococcal myositis, streptococcal bacteremia and streptococcal toxic shock syndrome (*3, 20, 22, 23*). These outbreaks have not been confined to socially and economically disadvantaged populations

Rheumatic fever and rheumatic heart disease

In 1994, it was estimated that 12 million individuals suffered from RF and RHD worldwide (*6*), and at least 3 million had congestive heart failure (CHF) that required repeated hospitalisation (*24*). A large proportion of the individuals with CHF required cardiac valve surgery within 5–10 years (*4, 6, 24*). The mortality rate for RHD varied from 0.5 per 100 000 population in Denmark, to 8.2 per 100 000 population in China (*25*), and the estimated annual number of deaths from RHD for 2000 was 332 000 worldwide (*26*). The mortality rate per 100 000 population varied from 1.8 in the WHO Region of the Americas, to 7.6 in WHO South-East Asia Region. The disability-adjusted life years (DALYs)[1] lost to RHD ranged from 27.4 DALYs per 100 000 population in the WHO Region of the Americas, to 173.4 per 100 000 population in the WHO South-East Asia Region. An estimated 6.6 million DALYs are lost per year worldwide (Table 2.2). Data from developing countries suggest that mortality due to RF and

---

[1] Disability-adjusted life years (DALYs) lost is the sum of years of life lost owing to premature death, plus the years lived with disability adjusted for the severity of the disability (*24*).

5

Table 2.2

Estimated deaths and DALYs lost to rheumatic heart disease in 2000, by WHO Region[a]

WHO Region	Deaths		DALYs[b] lost	
	N ($\times 10^3$)	Rate (per 100 000 population)	n ($\times 10^6$)	Rate (per 100 000 population)
Africa	29	4.5	0.77	119.8
The Americas	15	1.8	0.24	27.4
Eastern Mediterranean	21	4.4	0.59	121.6
Europe	38	4.3	0.49	56.1
South-East Asia	117	7.6	2.66	173.4
Western Pacific	115	6.8	1.78	105.4
World	332	5.5	6.63	109.6

[a] Source: 26.
[b] DALYs = disability-adjusted life years.

RHD remains a problem and that children and young adults still die from acute RF (*4–6, 14, 24–26*).

Reliable data on the incidence of RF are scarce. In some countries, however, local data obtained from RF registers of schoolchildren provide useful information on trends. The annual incidence of RF in developed countries began to decrease in the 20th century, with a marked decrease after the 1950s; it is now below 1.0 per 100 000 (*6*). A few studies conducted in developing countries report incidence rates ranging from 1.0 per 100 000 school-age children in Costa Rica (*27*), 72.2 per 100 000 in French Polynesia, 100 per 100 000 in Sudan, to 150 per 100 000 in China (*6*).

The prevalence of RHD has also been estimated in surveys, mainly of school-age children. The surveys results showed there was wide variation between countries, ranging from 0.2 per 1000 schoolchildren in Havana, Cuba, to 77.8 per 1000 in Samoa (Table 2.3; *1, 28–45*). The prevalence of RF and RHD and the mortality rates varied widely between countries and between population groups in the same country, such as between Maoris and non-Maoris in New Zealand, Samoans and Chinese in Hawaii, and Aboriginals and non-Aboriginals in Northern Australia (*1, 2, 5, 6, 12, 17*).

Although it is known that hospital morbidity data often give biased information about the magnitude of diseases, they are the only data available in many developing countries. Based on such data, RHD accounts for 12–65% of hospital admissions related to cardiovascular disease, and for 2.0–9.9% of all hospital discharges in some

Table 2.3
Examples of reported prevalence of rheumatic heart disease in schoolchildren

Source	WHO Region (country, city)	Year	Rate (per 1000 population)
	Africa		
28	Kenya (Nairobi)	1994	2.7
29	Zambia (Lusaka)	1986	12.5
30	Ethiopia (Addis Ababa)	1999	6.4
31	Conakry (Republic of Guinea)	1992	3.9
32	DR Congo (Kinshasa)	1998	14.3
	Americas		
33	Cuba (Havana, Santiago, P. del Rio)	1987	0.2–2.9
34	Bolivia (La Paz)	1986–1990	7.9
	Eastern Mediterranean		
35	Morocco	1989	3.3–10.5
34	Egypt (Cairo)	1986–1990	5.1
34	Sudan (Khartoum)	1986–1990	10.2
36	Saudi Arabia	1990	2.8
37	Tunisia	1990	3.0–6.0
	South-East Asia		
38	Northern India	1992–1993	1.9–4.8
39	India	1984–1995	1.0–5.4
40	Nepal (Kathmandu)	1997	1.2
41	Sri Lanka	1998	6
	Western Pacific		
1	Cook Islands	1982	18.6
1	French Polynesia	1985	8.0
42	New Zealand (Hamilton)	1983	6.5 (Maoris) 0.9 (non-Maoris)
45	Samoa	1999	77.8
43	Australia (Northern Territory)	1989–1993	9.6

developing countries (*5, 6, 46*). There has been a marked decrease in the mortality, incidence, prevalence, hospital morbidity and severity of RF and RHD in some places that have implemented prevention programmes, such as; Havana, Cuba; Costa Rica; Cairo, Egypt; and Martinique and Guadeloupe (*2, 5, 6, 27, 44, 47–54*).

Determinants of the disease burden of rheumatic fever and rheumatic heart disease

It is well known that socioeconomic and environmental factors play an indirect, but important, role in the magnitude and severity of RF and RHD. Factors such as a shortage of resources for providing quality health care, inadequate expertise of health-care providers,

Table 2.4
Direct and indirect results of environmental and health-system determinants on rheumatic fever and rheumatic heart disease

Determinants	Effects	Impact on RF and RHD burden
Socioeconomic and environmental factors: (poverty, undernutrition, overcrowding, poor housing).	Rapid spread of group A streptococcal strains. Difficulties in accessing health care.	Higher incidence of acute streptococcal-pharyngitis and suppurative complications. Higher incidence of acute RF. Higher rates of recurrent attacks.
Health-system related factors: — shortage of resources for health care; — inadequate expertise of health-care providers; — low-level awareness of the disease in the community.	Inadequate diagnosis and treatment of streptococcal pharyngitis. Misdiagnosis or late diagnosis of acute RF. Inadequate secondary prophylaxis and/or non-compliance with secondary prophylaxis.	Higher incidence of acute RF and its recurrence. Patients unaware of the first RF episode. More severe evolution of disease. Untimely initiation or lack of secondary prophylaxis. Higher rates of recurrent attacks with more frequent and severe heart valve involvement, and higher rates of repeated hospital admissions and expensive surgical interventions.

and a low level of awareness of the disease in the community can all impact the expression of the disease in populations. Crowding adversely affects rheumatic fever incidence (*1–7, 14, 22, 23*) (Table 2.4).

References

1. *Rheumatic fever and rheumatic heart disease. Report of a WHO Study Group.* Geneva, World Health Organization, 1988 (Technical Report Series, No. 764).

2. **Taranta A, Markowitz M.** *Rheumatic fever.* Boston, Kluwer Academic Publishers, **1989**:1–18.

3. **Kaplan E.** Recent epidemiology of Group A streptococcal infections in North America and abroad: an overview. *Pediatrics*, 1996, **97**(6): S945–S948.

4. World Health Report. *Conquering suffering. Enriching humanity.* Geneva, World Health Organization, 1997:43–44.

5. **KrishnaKumar R et al.** Epidemiology of streptococcal pharyngitis, rheumatic fever and rheumatic heart disease. In: Narula J et al., eds. *Rheumatic fever.* Washington, DC, American Registry of Pathology Publisher, 1999:41–78.

6. *Joint WHO/ISFC meeting on RF/RHD control with emphasis on primary prevention, Geneva, 7–9 September 1994.* Geneva, World Health Organization, 1994 (WHO Document WHO/CVD 94.1).

7. **Bisno AL.** Acute pharyngitis: etiology and diagnosis. *Pediatrics*, 1996, 97(6):S949–S954.

8. **Carapetis JR et al.** Epidemiology and prevention of group A streptococcal infection: acute respiratory tract infections, skin infections, and their sequelae at the close of the twentieth century. *Clinical Infectious Diseases*, 1999, 28:205–210.

9. **Shulman ST et al.** Streptococcal infections. In: Stevens D, Kaplan E, eds. *Clinical aspects, microbiology, and molecular pathogenesis.* New York, Oxford University Press, 2000:76–101.

10. **Kaplan EL.** The group A streptococcal upper respiratory tract carrier state: an enigma. *Journal of Pediatrics*, 1980, 97(3):337–345.

11. **Pruksakorn S et al.** Epidemiological analysis of non-M-typeable group A Streptococcus isolates from a Thai population in Northern Thailand. *Journal of Clinical Microbiology*, 2000, 38(3):1250–1254.

12. **Nandi S et al.** Group A streptococcal sore throat in a periurban population of Northern India: a one-year prospective study. *Bulletin of the World Health Organization*, 2001, 79:528–533.

13. **Begovac J et al.** Asymptomatic pharyngeal carriage of beta-haemolytic streptococci and streptococcal pharyngitis among patients at an urban hospital in Croatia. *European Journal of Epidemiology*, 1993, 9(4):405–410.

14. **Fraser GE.** A review of the epidemiology and prevention of rheumatic Heart disease: Part II. Features and epidemiology of streptococci. *Cardiovascular Review and Report*, 1996, 17(4):7–23.

15. **Nordet P et al.** Amigdalofaringitis aguda. Estudio clinico-bacteriologico y terapeutico. [Acute tonsilo-pharyngitis. Clinical, bacteriological and therapeutic study.] *Revista Cubana Pediatria, [Cuban Journal of Pediatrics,]* 1989, 61(6):821–833.

16. **Steihoff MC et al.** Effectiveness of clinical guidelines for the presumptive treatment of streptococcal pharyngitis in Egyptian children. *The Lancet*, 1997, 350:918–921.

17. **Dagnelie CF et al.** Bacterial flora in patients presenting with sore throat in Dutch general practice. *British Journal of General Practice*, 1998, 427:959–962.

18. **Cohen R et al.** Towards a better diagnosis of throat infections (with group A beta haemolytic streptococcus) in general practice. *British Journal of General Practice*, 1998, 427:959–962.

19. **Anthony BF et al.** The dynamics of streptococcal infections in a defined population of children: serotypes associated with skin and respiratory infections. *American Journal of Epidemiology*, 1976, 104:652–666.

20. **Kaplan EL et al.** Group A streptococcal serotypes isolated from patients and siblings contact during the resurgence of rheumatic fever in the United States in the mid-80s. *Journal of Infectious Diseases*, 1989, **159**:101–103.

21. **Veasy LG et al.** Persistence of acute rheumatic fever in the intermountain area of the United States. *Journal of Pediatrics*, 1994, **124**:9–16.

22. **Bronze MS, Dale JB.** The re-emergence of serious group A streptococcal infections and acute rheumatic fever. *American Journal of Medical Science*, 1996, **311**(1):41–54.

23. *The WHO Programme on Streptococcal Disease Complex. Report of a Consultation. Geneva, 16–19 February 1998.* Geneva, World Health Organization, 1998 (WHO document EMC/BAC/98.7).

24. **Murray CJ, Lopez AD, eds.** In: *Global health statistics.* Cambridge, Harvard University Press, 1996:64–67. (See also: Murray CJ, Lopez AD, eds. In: *Global burden of disease and injury series.* Cambridge, Harvard University Press, **1996**:643–645).

25. *World Health Statistical Annual 1990–2000.* Geneva, World Health Organization.

26. Health system: improving performance. In: *The World Health Report 2001.* Geneva, World Health Organization, **2001**:144–155.

27. **Arguedas A, Mohs E.** Prevention of rheumatic fever in Costa Rica. *Journal of Pediatrics*, 1992, **121**(4):569–572.

28. **Anabwani GM et al.** Prevalence of heart disease in school children in rural Kenya using colour-flow echocardiograph. *East African Medical Journal*, 1996, **73**(4):215–217.

29. **Mukelabai K et al.** Rheumatic heart disease in a sub-Saharan African city: epidemiology, prophylaxis and health education. *Cardiologie Tropicale, [Tropical Cardiology]* 2000, **26**(102):25–28.

30. **Oli K et al.** Prevalence of rheumatic heart disease among school children in Addis Ababa. *East African Medical Journal*, 1999, **76**(11):601–605.

31. **Toure S et al.** Enquête sur les cardiopaties en mielieu scolaire et universitaire ã Conakry, R. de Guinée. [Prevalence of cardiopathies in primary school, secondary school and university in Conakri, R. Guinéa.] *Cardiologie Tropicale, [Tropical Cardiology]* 1992, **18**(72):205–210.

32. **Longo-Mbenza et al.** Survey of rheumatic heart disease in schoolchildren of Kinshasa town. *International Journal of Cardiology*, 1998, **63**(3):287–294.

33. **Nordet P. et al.** Fiebre reumática en Cuba: incidencia, prevalencia, mortalidad y caracteristicas clinicas. [Rheumatic fever and rheumatic hear disease in Cuba: incidence, prevalence mortality and clinical characteristics.] *Revista Cubana de Cardiologia y Cirugia Cardiovascular, [Cuban Journal of Cardiology and Cardiovascular Surgery]* 1991, **5**(1):25–33.

34. WHO/CVD Unit. WHO programme for the prevention of rheumatic fever/ rheumatic heart disease in 16 developing countries (AGFUND). Report from Phase I (1986–1990). *Bulletin of the World Health Organization*, 1982, **70**(2):213–218.

35. *Le rhumatisme articulaire aigu: réalités et perspectives au Maroc*. L' Objectif médical, Edition Maroc. Numéro spécial et hors série, 1990.

36. **Al-Sekait MA et al.** Rheumatic fever and chronic rheumatic heart disease in schoolchildren in Saudi Arabia. *Saudi Medical Journal*, 1991, **12**:407–410.

37. **Kechrid A et al.** Acute rheumatic fever in Tunisia. In: Horoued et al., eds. *Streptococci and the host*. New York, Plenum Press Publishers, **1997**:121–123.

38. **Thakur JS et al.** Epidemiological survey of rheumatic heart disease among school children in the Shimla Hills of northern India: prevalence and risk factors. *Journal of Epidemiology and Community Health*, 1996, **50**(1):62–67.

39. **Padmavati S.** Rheumatic heart disease: prevalence and preventive measures in the Indian subcontinent. *Heart*, 2001, **86**:127.

40. **Prakash RR et al.** Prevalence of rheumatic fever and rheumatic heart disease in school children of Kathmandu city. *Indian Heart Journal*, 1997, **49**:518–520.

41. **Mendis S, Nasser M, Perera K.** A study of rheumatic heart disease and rheumatic fever in a defined population in Sri Lanka. *The Ceylon Journal of Medical Science*, 1998, **40**(2):31–37.

42. **Talbot RG.** Rheumatic fever and rheumatic heart disease in the Hamilton health district: an epidemiological survey. *New Zealand Medical Journal*, 1984, **97**:630–634.

43. **Carapetis JR et al.** Acute rheumatic fever and rheumatic heart disease in the top end of Australia's Northern Territory. *Medical Journal of Australia*, 1996, **164**(3):146–149.

44. **Nordet P. et al.** Fiebre reumatica in Ciudad de la Habana. Prevalencia y caracteristicas, 1972–1987. [Rheumatic fever in Havana. Prevalence and characteristics, 1972–1987.] *Revista Cubana Pediatria, [Cuban Journal of Pediatrics,]* 1989, **61**(2):228–237.

45. **Steer A.** Rheumatic heart disease in school children in Samoa. *Archives of Disease in Childhood*, 1999, **81**(4):373–374.

46. **Bertrand E.** Morbidité Cardiovasculaire en Afrique Subsaharienne en 1990–2000. [Cardiovascular morbidity in sub-Saharan Africa between 1990–2000.] *Cardiologie Tropicale, [Tropical Cardiology,]* 2000, **26**(104):88–89.

47. The WHO Global Programme for the prevention of RF/RHD. *Report of a consultation to review progress and develop future activities*. Geneva, World Health Organization, 2000 (WHO document WHO/CVD/00.1).

48. **Gordis L.** The virtual disappearance of rheumatic fever in the United States: lessons in the rise and fall of disease. *Circulation*, 1985, **72**(6):1155–1162.

49. **Strasser T et al.** The community control of rheumatic fever and rheumatic heart disease: report of a WHO international cooperative project. *Bulletin of the World Health Organization*, 1981, **59**(2):285–294.

50. **Flight RJ.** The Northland rheumatic fever register. *New Zealand Medical Journal*, 1984, **97**:671–673.

51. **Bach JF et al.** Ten-year educational programme aimed at rheumatic fever in two French Caribbean islands. *The Lancet*, 1996, **347**:644–648.

52. **Neilson G et al.** Rheumatic fever and chronic rheumatic heart disease in Yarrabah aboriginal community, North Queensland. Establishment of a prophylactic program. *Medical Journal of Australia*, 1993, **158**:316–318.

53. **Majeed, HA et al.** The natural history of acute rheumatic fever in Kuwait: a prospective six-year follow-up report. *Journal of Chronic Diseases*, 1986, **39**(5):361–369.

54. **Bitar FF et al.** Rheumatic fever in children: a 15-year experience in a developing country. *Pediatric Cardiology*, 2000, **21**(2):119–122.

3. Pathogenesis of rheumatic fever

Introduction

The epidemiological association between group A β-haemolytic streptococcal infections and the subsequent development of acute rheumatic fever (RF) has been well established. RF is a delayed autoimmune response to Group A streptococcal pharyngitis, and the clinical manifestation of the response and its severity in an individual is determined by host genetic susceptibility, the virulence of the infecting organism, and a conducive environment (*1–3*). Although streptococci from serogroups B, C, G and F can cause pharyngitis and trigger a host immune response, they have not been linked to the etiology of RF or rheumatic heart disease (RHD). There is considerable geographical variation in the prevalence of all serogroups of β-haemolytic streptococci. In many tropical countries, up to 60–70% of isolates from the throats of asymptomatic children fall into serogroups C and G. Conversely, in temperate regions, serogroup A is the predominant isolate (50–60%), with serogroups C and G together accounting for less than 30% of isolates. Nonsuppurative sequel, such as RF and RHD, are seen only after group A streptococcal infection of the upper respiratory tract. Post-streptococcal glomerulonephritis may occur after an infection of either the throat or skin by nephritogenic strains of group A streptococci (*1, 2*). It is presumed that chronic streptococcal "carrier" states do not trigger the development of RF (*1–5*).

Although substantial progress has been made in the understanding of RF as an autoimmune disease, the precise pathogenetic mechanism of RF has not been defined. Major histocompatibiltiy antigens, potential tissue-specific antigens, and antibodies developed during and immediately after a streptococcal infection are being investigated as potential risk factors in the pathogenesis of the disease. Recent evidence suggests that T-cell lymphocytes play an important role in the pathogenesis of rheumatic carditis. It has also been postulated that particular M types of group A streptococci have rheumatogenic potential. Such serotypes are usually heavily encapsulated, and form large, mucoid colonies that are rich in M-protein. These characteristics enhance the ability of the bacteria to adhere to tissue, as well as their ability to resist phagocytosis in the human host. However encapsulation is not exclusive to these strains and much of the data supporting the idea of selective "rheumatogenicity" is anecdotal (*1, 5*).

Streptococcal M-protein

M-protein is one of the best-defined determinants of bacterial virulence. The streptococcal M-protein extends from the surface of the streptococcal cell as an alpha–helical coiled coil dimer, and shares structural homology with cardiac myosin and other alpha-helical coiled coil molecules, such as tropomyosin, keratin and laminin. It has been suggested that this homology is responsible for the pathological findings in acute rheumatic carditis. Laminin, for example, is an extracellular matrix protein secreted by endothelial cells that line the heart valves and is an integral part of the valve structure. It is also a target for a polyreactive antibody that recognizes M-protein, myosin and laminin.

The M-protein molecule has a hypervariable N-terminal region, a conserved C-terminal region, and is divided into A, B and C repeat regions on the basis of peptide sequence periodicity (5–7). Epitopes that are cross-reactive in myocardium, synovia and brain are located between the B and C repeat regions, away from the type-specific epitopes in the N-terminal region. The C repeat regions contain highly conserved epitopes, and streptococci are often classified into Class I or II, based on whether their M-protein reacts with a monoclonal antibody (10B6) that targets epitopes in the C repeat region of the M6 molecule. The majority of Class I strains (with reactive M-protein) are implicated in RF. Of the more than 130 M-protein types identified, M types such as 1, 3, 5, 6, 14, 18, 19 and 24 have been associated with RF. However, not all M-protein serotypes are associated with RF and serotypes 2, 49, 57, 59, 60 and 61, for example, have been associated with pyoderma and acute glomerulonephritis (4, 5). Class II strains, on the other hand, have nonreactive M-proteins and produce an apolipoproteinase called opacity factor (7, 8). Individuals may have multiple streptococcal infections throughout their lifetime, but reinfections with the same serological M type are relatively less common because individuals acquire circulating homologous anti-M antibodies following an infection.

Streptococcal superantigens

Superantigens are a unique group of glycoproteins synthesized by bacteria and viruses that can bridge Class II major histocompatibility complex molecules to nonpolymorphic V β-chains of the T-cell receptors, simulating antigen binding. The T-cells bearing the appropriate V β-chain are activated (to release cytokines or become cytotoxic), regardless of their antigenic specificity. Some T-cells activated in this manner can have autoreactive specificities, since previously anergized T-cell subsets are susceptible to superantigenic stimulation. In the case of streptococci, much work has focused on the role of the superantigen-like activity of M-protein fragments (PeP M5, in particular), as well as the streptococcal pyrogenic exotoxin, in the pathogenesis of RF (*4, 5, 9, 10*).

Superantigenic activation is not limited to the T-cell compartment alone. Streptococcal erythrogenic toxin may behave like a superantigen for the B-cell, leading to the production of autoreactive antibodies, but as noted above, much of the evidence is still indirect. Progress in genetic studies, and the identification of extracellular products and cell-wall components represent advances in knowledge about the virulence of group A streptococci. The role of GRAB (an alpha-2 macroglobulin-binding protein expressed by *Streptococcus pyogenes*), streptococcal fibronectin-binding protein 1 (sfb1), which mediates streptococcal adherence and invasion into human epithelial cells, and streptococcal C5a peptidase (SCPA), which inactivates complement chemotaxin C5a and allows streptococci to adhere to tissues, are all subjects of active research in the pathogenesis of streptococcal infections. These studies have also facilitated the genotypic and phenotypic characterization of group A streptococcal strains (*3–8, 11–19*).

The role of the human host in the development of rheumatic fever and rheumatic heart disease

There is strong evidence that an autoimmune response to streptococcal antigens mediates the development of RF and RHD in a susceptible host. Genetically-programmed determinants of host susceptibility to RF have been studied extensively, in an attempt to determine why only 0.3–3% of individuals with acute streptococcal pharyngitis go on to develop RF (*1–3*). Pedigree studies suggested that this immune response is genetically controlled, with high responsiveness to the streptococcal cell-wall antigen being expressed through a single recessive gene, and low responsiveness through a single dominant gene. Further data indicate that the gene controlling the low-level response to streptococcal antigen is closely linked to the Class II human leukocyte antigen, HLA (*20*). However, studies of different HLA-DR loci and ethnicity further suggested that the link between susceptibility to RF and Class II HLA was highly diverse and not linked to one particular allele, but to a susceptibility gene present at, or nearby, the HLA-DR locus. For example, DR4 was present more frequently in Caucasian RF patients; DR2 more frequently in African-American populations (*21*); DR1 and DRw6 in RF patients from South Africa (*10*); and HLA-DR3 was present more frequently in RF patients in India (who also had a low frequency of DR2). In addition, DQW2 was present more frequently in Asian RF patients. Subsequently, it was reported that a B-lymphocyte alloantigen, recognized by the monoclonal antibody, D8/17, and another 70-kD molecule, may be genetically innate markers of an altered immune response to unidentified streptococcal antigens in susceptible subjects. The implication of an alloantigen on B-cells of patients with RF is currently being studied (1).

Host-pathogen interaction

Infection by streptococci begins with the binding of bacterial surface ligands to specific receptors on host cells, and subsequently involves specific processes of adherence, colonization and invasion. The binding of bacterial surface ligands to host surface receptors is the most crucial event in the colonization of the host, and it is initiated by fibronectin and by streptococcal fibronectin-binding proteins (17). Streptococcal lipoteichoic acid and M-protein also play a major role in bacterial adherence (9). The host responses to streptococcal infection include type-specific antibody production, opsonization and phagocytosis.

The role of environmental factors in RF and RHD

Secular trends in RF and RHD over the last one-and-a-half centuries, in both the developed and developing countries, all point towards environmental factors such as poor living conditions, overcrowding and access to health care as the most significant determinants of disease distribution (1–5). Indeed, the global distributions of RF and RHD are still influenced by socioeconomic indices, and the recent outbreak of RF in the USA is an aberration to this otherwise valid maxim. Crowded living conditions, with close interpersonal contacts, contribute to the rapid spread and persistence of virulent streptococcal strains. Seasonal variations in the incidence of RF (i.e. high incidences in early fall, late winter and early spring) closely mimic variations in streptococcal infections. These variations are particularly pronounced in temperate climates, but are not significant in the tropics.

Conclusions

It is evident from the preceding discussion that the pathogenesis of RF and RHD is a complex maze of events that are immunologically intricate, pathologically significant, and clinically devastating for the patients. It is ironic that a rather innocuous "sore throat" should extract such a high price from the host. As scientific research evolves, it is hoped that the gaps in our understanding will be filled, and better strategies for prophylaxis and treatment will become available. The following is a summary of our current understanding of the pathogenetic maze of rheumatic carditis.

Initial streptococcal infection in a genetically predisposed host in a susceptible environment leads to the activation of T-cell and B-cell lymphocytes by streptococcal antigens and superantigens, which results in the production of cytokines and antibodies directed against streptococcal carbohydrate and myosin. It has been proposed that injury to the valvular endothelium by the anti-carbohydrate antibodies leads to an up-regulation of VCAM1 and other adhesion molecules (10). VCAM1 expression is a hallmark of inflammation and it heralds cellular infiltration. VCAM1 interacts with VLA4 on activated lymphocytes and leads to an influx of activated CD4+ and CD8+ T-cells. A break in the endothelial continuity of a heart valve would expose subendothelial structures (vimentin, laminin and valvular interstitial cells) and lead to a "chain reaction" of valvular destruction. Once valve leaflets are inflamed through the valvular surface endothelium and new vascularization occurs, the newly formed microvasculature allows T-cells to infiltrate and perpetuate the cycle of valvular damage. The presence of T-cell infiltration, even in old mineralized lesions, is indicative of persistent and progressive disease in the valves. Valvular interstitial cells and other valvular constituents under the influence of inflammatory cytokines perpetuate aberrant repair.

Although the foregoing offers a very feasible explanation of the experimental data, questions remain that have significant implications for choosing streptococcal vaccines (22–24). For example, there is no direct and conclusive evidence for a pathogenetic role of cross-reactive antibodies *in vivo* and there is no exact animal model of rheumatic fever for study. The need for a better understanding of the epidemiology of streptococci is underscored by a report that one group A streptococcal serotype can be rapidly and completely replaced by another serotype in a stable population with adequate access to health care (25). This serotype change still has not been adequately explained and it raises questions about the efficacy of any type-specific streptococcal vaccine that is synthesized by combining M-protein sequences from virulent streptococcal serotypes. Furthermore, the ability of streptococci to infect the host after a prior infection by a different M serotype strain, suggests there is no broad, non-type-specific immunity directed against conserved M-protein epitopes or their extracellular products, which complicates the development of a RF vaccine aimed at conserved M-protein sequences.

The pathogenesis of RF will continue to perplex clinicians until such questions are answered.

References

1. *Rheumatic fever and rheumatic heart disease. Report of a WHO Study Group.* Geneva, World Health Organization, 1988 (Technical Report Series No. 764).

2. Kaplan EL. The group A streptococcal upper respiratory tract carrier state: an enigma. *Journal of Pediatrics*, 1980, **97**:337–339.

3. Taranta A, Markowitz M. *Rheumatic fever.* Boston, Kluwer Academic Publishers, 1989:19–25.

4. Narula J et al. *Rheumatic fever.* Washington, the American Registry of Pathology Publisher, 1999:48–68 and 103–194.

5. Stevens D, Kaplan E. *Streptococcal infections. Clinical aspects, microbiology and molecular pathogenesis.* New York, Oxford University Press, 2000:102–132.

6. Proft T et al. Identification and characterization of novel superantigens from *Streptococcus pyogenes. Journal of Experimental Medicine*, 1999, **189**:89–101.

7. Hallas G, Widdowson JP. The relationship between opacity factor and M protein in *Streptococcus pyogenes. Journal of Medical Microbiology*, 1983, **16**(1):13–26.

8. Widdowson JP et al. The relationship between M-antigen and opacity factor in group A streptococci. *Journal of General Microbiology*, 1971, **65**(1):69–80.

9. Kotb M, Watanabe-Ohnishi R, Wang B. Analysis of the TCR V beta specificities of bacterial superantigens using PCR. *Immunomethods*, 1993, **2**:33–40.

10. Roberts S et al. Pathogenic mechanisms in rheumatic carditis: focus on valvular endothelium. *Journal of Infectious Diseases,* 2001, **183**(3):507–511.

11. Swanson JE, Hsu KC, Gotschlich EC. Electron microscopic studies on streptococci IM antigen. *Journal of Experimental Medicine*, 1969, **130**:1063–1091.

12. Alouf JE. Streptococcal toxins (streptolysin O, streptolysin S, erythrogenic toxin). *Pharmacology and Therapeutics*, 1980, **11**:661–717.

13. Hoe N et al. Rapid molecular genetic subtyping of serotype M1 group A streptococcus strains. *Emerging Infectious Diseases*, 1999, **5**(2):254–263.

14. Kaplan EL. The resurgence of group A streptococcal infections. *European Journal of Clinical Microbiology and Infectious Diseases*, 1991, **10**:55–57.

15. Holm SE et al. Aspects of pathogenesis of serious group A streptococcal infections in Sweden. *Journal of Infectious Diseases*, 1988–1999, **166**: 31–37.

16. Chen C, Bormann N, Cleary PP. VirR and Mry are homologous trans-acting regulators of M protein and C5a peptidase expression in group A streptococci. *Molecular and General Genetics*, 1993, **241**(5–6):685–693.

17. Simpson WA, Courtney HS, Ofek I. Interactions of fibronectin with streptococci: the role of fibronectin as a receptor for *Streptococcus pyogenes*. *Reviews of Infectious Diseases*, 1987, **9**(Suppl 4):S351–359.

18. Podbielski A, Krebs B, Kaufhold A. Genetic variability of the emm-related gene of the large vir regulon of group A streptococci: potential intra- and intergenomic recombination events. *Molecular and General Genetics*, 1994, **243**(6):691–698.

19. Ferretti JJ et al. Complete genome sequence of an M1 strain of *Streptococcus pyogenes*. *Proceedings of the National Academy of Sciences (USA)*, 2001, **98**(8):4658–4663.

20. Sasazuki T et al. An HLA-linked immune suppression gene in man. *Journal of Experimental Medicine*, 1980, **152**(2 Pt 2):297s–313s.

21. Ayoub EM et al. Association of class II human histocompatibility leukocyte antigens with rheumatic fever. *Journal of Clinical Investigation*, 1986, **77**(6):2019–2026.

22. Bessen D, Fischetti VA. Synthetic peptide vaccine against mucosal colonization by group A streptococci. I. Protection against a heterologous M serotype with shared C repeat region epitopes. *Journal of Immunology*, 1990, **145**(4):1251–1256.

23. Markowitz M, Gerber MA, Kaplan EL. Treatment of streptococcal pharyngotonsillitis: reports of penicillin's demise are premature. *Journal of Pediatrics*, 1993, **123**(5):679–685.

24. Liao L et al. Antibody-mediated autoimmune myocarditis depends on genetically determined target organ sensitivity. *Journal of Experimental Medicine*, 1995, **181**(3):1123–1131.

25. Kaplan EL, Wotton JT, Johnson DR. Dynamic epidemiology of group A streptococcal serotypes associated with pharyngitis. *Lancet*, 2001, **358**(9290):1334–1337.

4. Diagnosis of rheumatic fever

Jones criteria for the diagnosis of rheumatic fever

The Jones criteria were introduced in 1944 as a set of clinical guidelines for the diagnosis of rheumatic fever (RF) and carditis (*1*). The clinical features of RF were divided into major and minor categories, based on the prevalence and specificity of manifestations (Figure 1). Major manifestations were least likely to lead to an improper diagnosis and included carditis, joint symptoms, subcutaneous nodules, and chorea. A history of RF or preexisting rheumatic heart disease (RHD) was considered to be a major criterion since RF tends to recur. Minor manifestations were considered to be suggestive, but not sufficient, for a diagnosis of RF. The minor manifestations comprised clinical findings (such as fever and erythema marginatum, abdominal pain, epistaxis and pulmonary findings), and laboratory markers of acute inflammation, such as leukocytosis (WBC), and elevated erythrocyte sedimentation rate (ESR) or C-reactive protein (CRP) (Figure 1). It was proposed that the presence of two major, or one major and

Figure 1
Changes in the Jones criteria following reviews from AHA and WHO

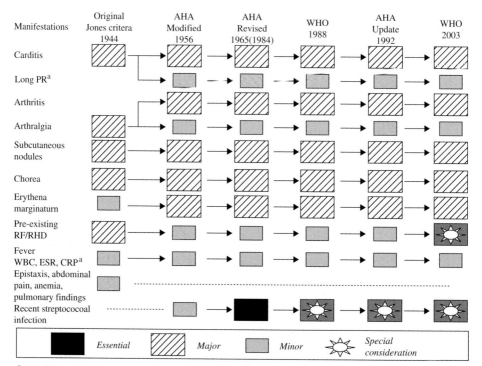

a PR = PR interval in the electrocardiogram; WBC = leukcoytosis; ESR = erythrocyteseyimontation rate; CRP = C-reactive protein.
Modified in part from reference (45)

two minor, manifestations offered reasonable clinical evidence of rheumatic activity. Since a previous history of definite RF or RHD was considered a major criterion, diagnosis of a recurrence of RF did not require strict application of these guidelines, and minor manifestations were considered sufficient for the diagnosis.

The importance of the Jones criteria was soon realized, especially as objective guidelines that allowed RF to be diagnosed uniformly in multicenter studies of RF. The Jones criteria were subsequently reviewed by the American Heart Association (AHA) and the World Health Organization (WHO) (2–6) and were modified to encompass vexing clinical issues and to improve the specificity (Figure 1). Although the Jones criteria have been revised repeatedly, the modifications were often made without prospective studies and were based on the perceived effects of previous revision(s).

The importance of a preceding streptococcal infection has been emphasized in subsequent revisions of the Jones criteria, in which a diagnosis of RF required the demonstration of streptococcal etiology (2, 3). Although the inclusion of this criterion helped to improve diagnostic specificity, it impaired sensitivity when evidence of antecedent streptococcal infection had already subsided (such as with insidious and chronic carditis), or if manifestations of RF were delayed (such as with chorea) (7). Therefore, late manifestations of RF were subsequently exempted from the requirement to demonstrate streptococcal etiology (4, 5).

Carditis is the single most important prognostic factor in RF; only valvulitis leads to permanent damage and its presence determines the prophylactic strategy (8). The prophylactic and prognostic stakes clearly underscore the importance of correctly identifying carditis. The clinical diagnosis of carditis in an index attack of RF is based on the presence of significant murmurs (suggestive of mitral and/or aortic regurgitation), pericardial rub, or an unexplained cardiomegaly with CHF. Rheumatic cardiac involvement almost invariably occurs in an RF recurrence, if the initial episode involved the heart (9, 10). A diagnosis of recurring carditis requires the demonstration of valvular damage or involvement, with or without pericardial or myocardial involvement (11). Such clinical findings include a documented change in a previous murmur to a new murmur or pericardial rub, or an obvious radiographic increase in cardiac size, respectively. The clinical diagnosis of rheumatic carditis by the Jones criteria occasionally becomes difficult (9, 12, 13), such as during RF recurrence, especially when carditis is the sole manifestation of rheumatic activity. During a recurrence of rheumatic activity in a patient with preexisting RHD, the carditis may result in florid CHF, but it may not be possible to diagnose carditis from an interval change in valvular regurgitation owing to a lack of previous cardiac findings. This is in contrast to the primary RF episode, where unexplained CHF is considered sufficient for the diagnosis of active rheumatic carditis by the revised Jones criteria. It is important to differentiate between the recurrence of carditis as the cause of CHF, and the decompensation of chronic progressive valvular disease, because the use of steroids may be life-saving in active carditis, but of no benefit in valvular disease. The recurrent carditis is likely to remain subclinical in the absence of CHF and its diagnosis becomes even more difficult when previous cardiac findings are not known.

The majority of RF cases are observed in developing countries (*14*). Further, recurrences of the disease are common in developing countries, owing to gaps in the detection and secondary prevention of disease caused by a lack of health-care facilities. In such countries, the majority of active RF patients present with a recurrence of disease at least in the tertiary care setting.

2002–2003 WHO criteria for the diagnosis of rheumatic fever and rheumatic heart disease (based on the revised Jones criteria[3,4])

These revised WHO criteria (Table 4.1) facilitate the diagnosis of:

— a primary episode of RF
— recurrent attacks of RF in patients **without** RHD
— recurrent attacks of RF in patients **with** RHD
— rheumatic chorea
— insidious onset rheumatic carditis
— chronic RHD.

For the diagnosis of a primary episode of RF, it is recommended that the major and minor clinical manifestations of RF, the laboratory manifestations, and evidence of a preceding streptococcal infection should all continue according to the 1988 WHO recommendations (*6*). In the context of a preceding streptococcal infection, two major manifestations, or a combination of one major and two minor manifestations, provide reasonable evidence for a diagnosis of RF. WHO has continued to maintain that a diagnosis of a recurrence of RF in a patient with established RHD should be permitted on the basis of minor manifestations plus evidence of a recent streptococcal infection.

Physicians should use their clinical judgment to diagnose carditis in an episode of RF, especially during a recurrence of RF, and should use the above recommendations as guidelines for the diagnosis.

Table 4.1

2002–2003 WHO criteria for the diagnosis of rheumatic fever and rheumatic heart disease (based on the revised Jones criteria[3,4])

Diagnostic categories	Criteria
Primary episode of RF.[a]	Two major *or one major and two minor** manifestations **plus** evidence of a preceding group A streptococcal infection***.
Recurrent attack of RF in a patient **without** established rheumatic heart disease.[b]	Two major or one major and two minor manifestations **plus** evidence of a preceding group A streptococcal infection.
Recurrent attack of RF in a patient **with** established rheumatic heart disease.	Two minor manifestations **plus** evidence of a preceding group A streptococcal infection.[c]
Rheumatic chorea. Insidious onset rheumatic carditis.[b]	Other major manifestations or evidence of group A streptococcal infection not required.
Chronic valve lesions of RHD (patients presenting for the first time with pure mitral stenosis or mixed mitral valve disease and/or aortic valve disease).[d]	Do not require any other criteria to be diagnosed as having rheumatic heart disease.

* Major manifestations	— carditis — polyarthritis — chorea — erythema marginatum — subcutaneous nodules
** Minor manifestations	— clinical: fever, polyarthralgia — laboratory: elevated acute phase reactants (erythrocyte sedimentation rate or leukocyte count)
*** Supporting evidence of a preceding streptococcal infection within the last 45 days	— electrocardiogram: prolonged P-R interval — elevated or rising antistreptolysin-O or other streptococcal antibody, or — a positive throat culture, or — rapid antigen test for group A streptococci, or — recent scarlet fever.

[a] Patients may present with polyarthritis (or with only polyarthralgia or monoarthritis) and with several (3 or more) other minor manifestations, together with evidence of recent group A streptococcal infection. Some of these cases may later turnout to be rheumatic fever. It is prudent to consider them as cases of "probable rheumatic fever" (once other diagnoses are excluded) and advise regular secondary prophylaxis. Such patients require close follow up and regular examination of the heart. This cautious approach is particularly suitable for patients in vulnerable age groups in high incidence settings.
[b] Infective endocarditis should be excluded.
[c] Some patients with recurrent attacks may not fulfil these criteria.
[d] Congenital heart disease should be excluded.

Currently, clinical examination remains the basis of a diagnosis of RF and carditis, and the role of echocardiography should be considered supportive. However, an echo-Doppler examination should be performed if the facilities are available. The other invasive and noninvasive diagnostic modalities for RF, such as endomyocardial biopsy and radionuclide imaging, should be considered research tools.

Such recommendations are in keeping with the original intent of the Jones criteria, which were established as a universal standard for the diagnosis of RF.

Arthritis, chorea, erythema marginatum, and subcutaneous nodules are among the noncarditic manifestations considered to be major diagnostic features of acute RF. Subcutaneous nodules are almost always associated with cardiac involvement and are found more commonly in patients with severe carditis. Unlike rheumatic carditis, noncarditic manifestations of RF do not lead to permanent damage. The major noncarditic manifestations occur in varying combinations, with or without carditis, during the evolution of the disease. Arthritis is the most common manifestation of RF and usually draws attention to the disease. When arthritis appears as the sole major manifestation the clinical diagnosis of RF is difficult, because many infectious, immunological and vasculitic disorders may present with polyarthritis. The presence of noncarditic manifestations facilitates the detection of rheumatic carditis and their identification is particularly important in recurrences of disease, when the diagnosis of carditis is difficult.

Recently, techniques for detecting pericardial, myocardial and valvular involvement in RF have been studied (15), and WHO carefully reviewed their role in the diagnosis of RF, with special emphasis on their applicability in developing countries.

Diagnosis of rheumatic carditis

Although the endocardium, myocardium and pericardium are all affected to varying degrees, rheumatic carditis is almost always associated with a murmur of valvulitis (Table 4.2). Accordingly, myocarditis and pericarditis, by themselves, should not be labeled rheumatic in origin, when not associated with a murmur and other etiologies must be considered.

Valvulitis/endocarditis

A first episode of rheumatic carditis should be suspected in a patient who does not have a history suggestive of previous RF or RHD, and who develops a new apical systolic murmur of mitral regurgitation (with or without an apical mid-diastolic murmur), and/or the basal early diastolic murmur of aortic regurgitation. On the other hand, in an individual with previous RHD, a definite change in the character of any of these murmurs or the appearance of a new significant murmur indicates the presence of carditis.

Table 4.2
Clinical features of rheumatic carditis

Pericarditis: Audible friction rub; can be supported by echocardiographic evidence of pericardial effusion. Simultaneous demonstration of valvular involvement generally considered essential. Pericarditis is equally diagnostic in primary episode, or a recurrence of RF.

Myocarditis: Unexplained CHF or cardiomegaly, almost always associated with valvular involvement. Left ventricular function is rarely affected. In presence of RHD, CHF and minor manifestations, and elevated streptococcal antibody titers provide reasonable evidence of rheumatic carditis.

Endocarditis/valvulitis: Presence of apical holosystolic murmur of mitral regurgitation (with or without apical mid-diastolic murmur, Carey Coombs), or basal early diastolic murmur in patients who do not have a history of RHD.

On the other hand, in an individual with previous RHD, a definite change in the character of any of these murmurs or the appearance of a new significant murmur indicates the presence of carditis.

Echocardiography[a] can provide early evidence of valvular involvement, can confirm suspected valvular regurgitation, and can exclude non-rheumatic causes of valvular involvement.

---

[a] Echocardiographic demonstration of valvular regurgitation is not a prerequisite for the diagnosis of rheumatic carditis and should not be considered a limitation where the facilities are not available. The strict application of diagnostic criteria is mandatory to demonstrate pathological valvular regurgitation. Currently, data do not allow subclinical valvular regurgitation detected by echocardiography to be included in the Jones criteria, as evidence of a major manifestation of carditis. Echocardiography can only play a limited role in cases of recurring RF, unless a previous echocardiographic study is available for comparison.

Myocarditis

Myocarditis (alone) in the absence of valvulitis is unlikely to be of rheumatic origin and by itself should not be used as a basis for such a diagnosis. It should always be associated with an apical systolic or basal diastolic murmur. Clinically apparent CHF and radiographic cardiac enlargement indicate that the myocardium is likely to be involved in the primary episode of RF, although the role of unexplained CHF in the diagnosis of a recurrence of rheumatic carditis has been questioned. It seems safe to recommend that an unexplained worsening of CHF in a suspected case of recurrent RF indicates the presence of active carditis, if supported by adequate minor manifestations and evidence of a preceding streptococcal infection. If previous clinical findings are known, they can be compared with current data — myocardial involvement is likely to result in a sudden cardiac enlargement that will be detectable radiographically. Infective endocarditis may also masquerade as a recurrence of rheumatic fever.

Patients with CHF are considered to suffer from severe carditis. Although CHF has always been directly linked with myocardial involvement in RF, the impairment in left ventricular systolic function does not occur in RF, and the signs and symptoms of CHF may result from severe valvular incompetence (*16, 17*).

Pericarditis

Pericardial involvement in RF may result in distant heart sounds, a friction rub, and chest pain. At times, however, the friction rub can mask the mitral regurgitation murmur, which becomes evident only after the pericarditis subsides. Since isolated pericarditis is not good evidence of rheumatic carditis without supporting evidence of a valvular regurgitant murmur, it may be helpful to have Doppler echocardiography available in such circumstances to look for signs of mitral regurgitation. Echocardiography could also corroborate the mild-to-moderate pericardial effusion likely to be associated with pericarditis; large effusions and tamponade are rare (*18*). Although not specific, the electrocardiogram may show low-voltage QRS complexes and ST-T changes, and the heart may appear enlarged in an X-ray silhouette. Patients with this form of pericarditis are usually treated as cases of severe carditis.

Diagnosis of extra cardiac manifestations of RF

Although the cardiac manifestations of RF are most important in terms of immediate and long-term prognoses, the generalized inflammatory process in RF, as defined in the 1988 WHO revision of the Jones Criteria (*6*), may occur in extra cardiac target sites (e.g. skin, joints, brain) during the evolution of the disease. Noncardiac manifestations may be the best guide for a diagnosis of rheumatic carditis. As with previous editions of the Jones Criteria, the presence of two major criteria, or of one major and two minor criteria, indicates a high probability of RF, if supported by evidence of a prior Group A streptococcal infection. Absence of the latter always makes a diagnosis of RF doubtful, except for specific situations (Table 4.1).

Major manifestations
Arthritis

Arthritis is the most frequent major manifestation of RF, occurring in up to 75% of patients in the first attack of RF (*19, 20*). It occurs early in the course of the disease, as the presenting complaint. Arthritis is often the only major manifestation in adolescents, as well as in adults, where carditis and chorea become less common in older age groups. The involvement of joints in RF may present as arthralgia, to disabling arthritis. Joint pain without objective findings does not qualify as a major disease manifestation because of its nonspecificity. The articular manifestations in RF typically present as migratory poly-arthritis, most often in the larger joints (commonly in the knees and ankles); the wrists, elbows, shoulders and hips are less frequently involved; and the small joints of the hands, feet and neck are rarely affected (*20*). Inflamed joints are characteristically warm, red and swollen, and an aspirated sample of synovial fluid may reveal a high average leukocyte count (29 000 mm^{-3}, range 2000–96 000 mm^{-3}) (*21*). Tenderness in rheumatic arthritis may be out of proportion to the objective findings and severe enough to result in excruciating pain on touch. The term "migratory" reflects the sequential involvement of joints, with each completing a cycle of inflammation and resolution, so that some joint inflammation may be resolving while others are beginning.

Not all cases of rheumatic arthritis conform to this characteristic description. Monoarthritis may occur, for example, and its frequency increases when anti-inflammatory therapy is initiated before RF is fully expressed. Frequently, several joints may be affected simulta-neously, or the arthritis may be additive rather than migratory. In-flammation in a particular joint usually resolves within two weeks and the entire bout of polyarthritis in about a month if untreated.

Relation to other manifestations. Polyarthritis and Sydenham's chorea virtually never occur simultaneously due to the disparity in the la-tency period following the antecedent streptococcal infection. Chorea may, however, occur after arthritis has subsided. Carditis and arthritis frequently coexist during an RF episode, and demonstrate an inverse relationship between the severity of arthritis and carditis. One study, for example, found severe cardiac involvement in 10% of those with arthritis, 33% of those with arthralgia, and 50% of those with no joint symptoms (*19*).

Poststreptococcal reactive arthritis. Following a streptococcal infec-tion, some patients develop arthropathy that differs from acute rheu-matic arthritis. This entity, poststreptococcal arthritis, occurs after a relatively short latency period of about a week, may be persistent or relapsing (*22, 23*), may not respond dramatically to anti-inflammatory agents, and is not associated with other major manifestations of RF. It remains unclear whether it represents a form of reactive arthritis distinct from true RF, which may have important implications regard-ing prognosis and the need for antistreptococcal prophylaxis. A num-ber of patients presenting initially as poststreptococcal arthritis have later manifested RHD (*24*). Given our inability to differentiate be-tween a "benign" poststreptococcal arthritis and RF, patients with arthritis following a streptococcal upper respiratory infection should be considered to have RF if they fulfill the Jones criteria.

Differential diagnosis. Polyarthritis unaccompanied by other major manifestations of RF deserves differential diagnosis from many clinical entities (Tables 4.3 and 4.4) (*25*). Septic arthritis should be ruled out by microbiological studies. Gonococcal arthritis can present a problem because it occurs frequently in adolescents who do not have localized gonococcal disease, and whose blood and joint fluid cultures are negative in microbiological tests. The diagnosis can be helped by an epidemiological history and characteristic gonococcal skin lesions (if present), in addition to gonococcal cultures of urethra, cervix, rectum and pharynx.

Table 4.3
Differential diagnosis of polyarthritis and fever[a]

Diagnosis	Confirmatory study
Infectious arthritis	
Bacterial infections	
Septic arthritis	Synovial fluid and blood culture
Bacterial endocarditis	Blood culture
Lyme disease	Serological studies
Mycobacterial and fungal arthritis	Culture or biopsy
Viral arthritis	Serological studies
Postinfectious or reactive arthritis	
Enteric infection	Culture or serological studies
Urogenital infection (Reiter's syndrome)	Culture
RF	Clinical findings
Inflammatory bowel disease	Clinical findings
Rheumatoid arthritis and Still's disease	Clinical findings
Systemic rheumatic Illnesses	
Systemic vasculitis	Biopsy or angiography
Systemic lupus erythematosus	Serological studies
Crystal-induced arthritis	
Gout and pseudogout	Polarizing microscopy of synovial fluid or tophi
Other diseases	
Familial Mediterranean fever	Clinical findings
Cancers	Biopsy
Sarcoidosis	Biopsy
Mucocutaneous disorders	Biopsy or clinical findings
dermatomyositis	
Bechcet's disease	
Henoch-Schonlein purpura	
Kawasaki's disease (mucocutaneous lymph node syndrome)	
erythema nodosum	
erythema multiforme	
pyoderma gangrenosum	

[a] Source: (*25*).

Table 4.4
Discriminating features in patients presenting with polyarthritis and fever[a]

Symptom or sign	Possible diagnosis
Temperature of 40 °C	Still's disease Bacterial arthritis Systemic lupus eythematosus
Fever preceding arthritis	Viral arthritis Lyme disease Reactive arthritis Stills disease Bacterial endocarditis
Migratory arthritis	RF Gonococcemia Meningococcermia Viral arthritis Systemic lupus erythematosus Acute leukemia Whipple's disease
Effusion disproportionately greater than pain	Tuberculosis arthritis Bacterial endocarditis Inflammatory bowel disease Giant cell arthritis Lyme disease
Pain disproportionately greater than effusion	RF Familial Mediterranean fever Acute leukemia AIDS
Positive test for rheumatoid factor	Rheumatoid arthritis Viral arthritis Tuberculous arthritis Bacterial endocarditis Systemic lupus erythematosus Sarcoidosis Systemic vasculitis
Morning stiffness	Rheumatoid arthritis Polymyalgia rheumatica Still's disease Some viral and reactive arthritides
Symmetric small joint synovitis	Rheumatoid arthritis Systemic lupus erythematosus Viral arthritis
Leukocytosis (15 000 per mm^3)	Bacterial arthritis Bacterial endocarditis Still's disease Systemic vasculitis Acute leukemia
Leukopenia	Systemic lupus erythematosus Viral arthritis

Table 4.4
Continued

Symptom or sign	Possible diagnosis
Episodic recurrences	Lyme disease
	Crystal-induced arthritis
	Inflammatory bowel disease
	Whipple's disease
	Mediterranean fever
	Still's disease
	Juvenil Rheumatoid arthritis
	Systemic lupus erythematosus

[a] Source: (25).

Arthritis may also occur in infective endocarditis, and it may be difficult to differentiate this disease from RF, particularly when the endocarditis occurs in a patient with known RHD. The epidemiological features, history, physical examination, results of blood cultures, echocardiographic studies, and antistreptococcal antibody assays may all help to differentiate between infective endocarditis and RF. Lyme disease, which presents with arthritis, cardiac involvement, and skin lesions, may at times suggest RF; even the skin lesions of erythema chronicum migrans may resemble erythema marginatum. A diagnosis of Lyme disease should take into account the season of the year, geographical locale, and history of tick bites. The diagnosis can be confirmed by serological studies and the patient response to antimicrobial therapy.

Viremias, some of which are associated with immune complex formation, may also mimic rheumatic polyarthritis. Examples include hepatitis B and C, and rubella. Rheumatological manifestations of other immune complex diseases such as serum sickness may be confusing, particularly when they occur in a patient who has recently received antibiotics for an upper respiratory tract infection.

Finally, collagen vascular diseases, such as rheumatoid arthritis and systemic lupus erythematosus (SLE) may, at their onset, mimic RF. In juvenile rheumatoid arthritis certain associated findings, such as rash, lymphadenopathy and splenomegaly, may suggest the diagnosis. The cervical spine may also be involved in this disease, but is unusual in RF. At times, the only way to arrive at a definite diagnosis is to observe the clinical course. In addition, Henoch-Schonlein purpura, sickle-cell anemia, acute leukemia and gout at times mimic the arthritis of RF.

Prognosis. Arthritis heals completely, unlike carditis, and leaves no pathological or functional residua. The one possible exception is Joccoud chronic postrheumatic arthritis. This rare condition is not a true synovitis, but rather is a periarticular fibrosis of the metacarpophalangeal joints. It usually occurs in patients with severe RHD, but is not associated with evidence of RF (*26*).

Sydenham's chorea

Chorea occurs primarily in children and is rare after the age of 20 years. It occurs primarily in females, and almost never occurs in postpubertal males. The prevalence of chorea in RF patients varied from 5–36% in different reports (*27*). The reasons for the variation were not apparent, but might be related to differences in susceptibility to chorea in the host population, or to differences in case-finding methods. It is unknown whether particular strains of group A streptococci vary in their propensity to elicit chorea.

Sydenham's chorea is characterized by emotional lability, uncoordinated movements, and muscular weakness (*28, 29*). The onset may often be difficult to determine, as initially the child may become fretful, irritable, inattentive to schoolwork, fidgety, or even severely disturbed. Physical uncoordination soon becomes apparent, perhaps manifested as clumsiness and a tendency to drop objects, which progresses to spasmodic, uncoordinated movements. On physical examination, the movements are abrupt and erratic. All muscle groups may be affected, but erratic movements of the hands, feet and face are most evident. Facial movements include grimaces, grins and frowns. When the tongue is protruded it resembles a "bag of worms," and speech is jerky and staccato. Handwriting becomes illegible, and the patient may stumble when attempting to walk. When the hands are extended, the dorsum assumes a "spoon" or "dish" configuration due to flexion of the wrist and hyperextension of the metacarpophalangeal joints. When raising the hands above the head, the patient may pronate one or both hands ("pronator sign"). Patients with chorea are unable to sustain a titanic contraction; therefore, when asked to grip the examiner's hand, their irregular, repetitive squeezes have been termed "milkmaid grip". Although the choreiform movements are usually bilateral, they may be unilateral (hemichorea) (*30*). The choreiform movements disappear during sleep, decrease with rest and sedation, and can be suppressed by volition for few movements. They may be accentuated by asking the patient to perform several voluntary movements at once. Neither sensory deficits nor pyramidal tract involvement are present.

Relation to other manifestations of RF. Chorea may occur alone ("pure" chorea), or in association with other manifestations of RF. The relationship of chorea to polyarthritis and carditis was clarified by the recognition that chorea has a longer latency period after antecedent group A streptococcal infection, as long as 1–7 months. As a result, polyarthritis and Sydenham's chorea do not occur together; and indeed the onset of chorea often calls attention to subclinical carditis. Another consequence of the long latency period is that streptococcal antibody titres and laboratory measures of inflammation may have resolved by the time choreiform movements appears.

Choreic recurrences. Recurrent attacks of acute RF tend to be mimetic, and recurrences of chorea are not uncommon. As discussed above, when patients experience recurrent attacks of pure chorea, a preceding streptococcal infection may be difficult to establish. Frequently, patients with chorea gravidarum, or with oral contraceptive-induced chorea, have a past history of chorea (including Sydenham's chorea), suggesting that certain individuals may have an innate choreiform diathesis, or that a first attack confers an enhanced susceptibility to subsequent attacks.

Berrios et al. (*31*) observed 17 recurrences of pure chorea in 10 patients over a $5\frac{1}{2}$-year period. All patients were highly compliant with the prophylactic regimen and were followed prospectively, with monthly throat cultures and serum antistreptococcal antibody determinations every three months. In most cases, a recent streptococcal infection was confirmed by serological evidence, although titre increases were often quite modest. In four recurrences it was possible to rule out an immunologically significant streptococcal infection within the six months preceding the episode. It was concluded either that some recurrences of Sydenham's chorea in patients on optimal prophylaxis were triggered by streptococcal infections too weak and transient to be detected, or that stimuli other than streptococcal infections triggered the recurrences.

Differential diagnosis. In only approximately two-thirds of cases of pure chorea can a recent streptococcal infection be documented, which makes differential diagnosis more difficult. Non-cardiac chorea can occur owing to other collagen vascular, endocrine, metabolic, neoplastic, genetic, and infectious disorders (Table 4.5), perhaps the most common of which is SLE. It is not unusual for the central nervous system to be involved in SLE, and less than 2% of patients manifest chorea (*32*). The differentiation of SLE and RF is complicated by the occurrence of fever, arthritis, carditis, and skin lesions in both disorders.

Table 4.5
Guide to the differential diagnosis of chorea in children and adolescents[a]

Diagnosis	Diagnostic clues
Atypical seizure	Electroencephalographic abnormalities. Change in level of consciousness.
Cerebrovascular accidents	MRI[b] or CT evidence of lesion.
Collagen vascular disease (e.g. SLE, periarteritis nodosa)	History and physical examination. Laboratory evidence (e.g., decreased complement levels, positive ANA titers). (Note: ANA can be elevated following infection and therefore may be positive in acute RF).
Drug intoxication	Drug screen, especially for phenytoin, amitriptyline, metoclopramide, and fluphenazine.
Familiar chorea	The prototype is Huntington's disease, but the diagnosis also includes benign familial chorea, familial paroxysmal dystonic choreoathetosis, familial paroxysmal kinesigenic choreoathetosis, familial chorea with canthocytosis (check blood smear for acanthocytes), familial calcification of basal ganglia (MRI or CT scan may be helpful), ataxia telangiectasia, and Hallervorden-Spatz disease.
Hormonally induced chorea	Use of oral contraceptives. Pregnancy (chorea gravidarum)
Hyperthyroidism	Abnormal thyroid function test results.
Hypoparathyroidism	Low serum calcium and magnesium levels. High serum phosphorus level
Lyme disease	History and accompanying symptoms. Physical examination findings (e.g. rash) Titres against *Borrelia burgdorferi*
Sydneyham's chorea	Other signs of RF. Evidence of preceding streptococcal infection
Wilson's disease	Decreased serum ceruloplasmin level. Increased urinary copper excretion Kayser-Fleischer rings Anemia, hepatitis Family history

[a] Source: (*73*).
[b] Abbreviations: ANA = antinuclear antibody; CT = computed tomography; MRI = magnetic resonance imaging; SLE = systemic lupus erythematosus.

The occurrence of chorea during pregnancy, or chorea gravidarum, may remit prior to delivery or soon after. Because many of the patients have a history or prior attacks of chorea, it has been postulated that chorea gravidarum might represent a recurrence of RF during pregnancy. It is more likely, however, that in most cases the disorder is related to hormonal alterations. The role of hormonal factors in the pathogenesis of chorea is further exemplified by the association of choreic disorder associated with oral contraceptive use (33, 34). Chorea usually begins soon after the patient has started taking oral contraceptives and stops within a few weeks after they are discontinued. The manifestations are usually asymmetric or unilateral. Nearly half the patients have a history of previous chorea, which may have been associated with a rheumatic attack or with nonrheumatic conditions (e.g. chorea gravidarum, Henoch-Schonlein purpura). Interestingly, patients with oral contraceptive-induced chorea who later became pregnant do not necessarily develop chorea gravidarum. The pathogenesis of oral contraceptive-induced chorea remains obscure.

In addition to the above-mentioned causes of choreiform movements, simple motor tics in children or the involuntary jerks of Tourette's syndrome may be confused with chorea. However, the confounding feature is that many such disorders may also be secondary to the antecedent streptococcal infection, and collectively they have been referred to as PANDAS syndrome. However, at the present time, the PANDAS syndrome remains only an hypothesis and is not a proven entity.

Prognosis. The duration of chorea is quite variable, ranging from one week to more than two years; the median duration of an attack was 15 weeks in hospitalized patients. Three-quarters of the patients recover within six months. The manifestations of chorea may wax and wane during its course. A number of long-term neurological and psychological sequelae have been described, including convulsions, decreased learning ability, behavior problems, and psychosis. The exact relationship, if any, of these conditions to chorea is uncertain.

Subcutaneous nodules

The incidence of subcutaneous nodules in patients with RF varies widely in different studies and from country to country. The lesions have been reported in up to 20% of cases (35). The subcutaneous nodules are round, firm, freely movable, painless lesions varying in size from 0.5–2.0 cm. Because the skin over them is not inflamed, they may easily be missed if not carefully sought on physical examination. They occur in corps over bony prominences or extensor tendons. Common locations are the elbows, wrists, knees, ankles and Achilles tendons. They may also be found over the scalp, especially the occiput, and the spinous processes of the vertebrae. The number of nodules varies from one to a few dozen, but usually three or four. They persist from days to 1–2 weeks to, rarely, more than a month. The nodules are not pathognomonic of RF; similar lesions occur in SLE and rheumatoid arthritis. The nodules in the latter condition tend to be larger than those seen in RF.

Relation to other manifestations of RF. Subcutaneous nodules rarely occur as an isolated manifestation of RF. In most cases, they are associated with the presence of carditis, usually appearing several weeks after the onset of cardiac findings. Nodules are found more frequently in patients with severe carditis and may appear in recurrent corps (*36*).

Erythema marginatum

Erythema marginatum occurs in up to 15% of RF patients, although it was seen in only 4% of 274 patients admitted to the Primary Children's Medical Center in Salt Lake City, Utah, between 1985–1992 (*37*), and in 4% of 73 RF patients studied at the King Khalid University Hospital in Riyadh, Saudi Arabia, between 1985–1989 (*38*). In view of the evanescent nature of the lesions and the lack of associated symptoms, however, erythema marginatum may be missed if not specifically sought, particularly in dark-skinned patients.

The lesions of erythema marginatum appear first as a bright pink macule or papule that spreads outward in a circular or seripiginous pattern. The lesions are multiple, appearing on the trunk or proximal extremities, rarely on the distal extremities, and never on the face. They are nonpruritic and nonpainful, blanch under pressure, and are only rarely raised. Individual lesions may come and go in minutes to hours, at times changing shape before the observer's eye or coalescing with adjacent lesions to form varying patterns. Indeed, they have been described as appearing like "smoke rings" beneath the skin. Erythema marginatum usually occurs early in the course of a rheumatic attack. It may, however, persist or recur for months or even years, continuing after other manifestations of the disease have subsided, and it is not influenced by anti-inflammatory therapy. This cutaneous phenomenon is associated with carditis but, unlike subcutaneous nodules, not necessarily with severe carditis. Nodules and erythema marginatum tend to occur together.

Differential diagnosis. Erythema marginatum is not unique to RF and has also been reported during sepsis, drug reactions, and glomerulonephritis, and in children in whom no etiology is evident. It must be differentiated from other toxic erythemas in febrile patients and the rash of juvenile rheumatoid arthritis. The circinate rash of Lyme disease (erythema chronicum migrans) may resemble erythema marginatum.

Minor manifestations

Arthralgia and fever are termed "minor" clinical manifestations of RF in the Jones diagnostic criteria, not necessarily because they occur less frequently than the five recognized major criteria, but rather because they lack diagnostic specificity. Fever occurs in almost all rheumatic attacks at the onset, usually ranging from 101 °F to 104 °F (38.4–40.0 °C). Diurnal variations are common, but there is no characteristic fever pattern. Children who present only with mild carditis without arthritis may have a low-grade fever, and patients with pure chorea are afebrile. Fever rarely lasts more than several weeks. Arthralgia without objective findings is common in RF. The pain usually involves large joints, may be mild or incapacitating, and may be present for days to weeks, often varying in severity.

Although abdominal pain and epistaxis may occur in only about 5% of patients with RF, they have not been considered a part of the Jones criteria owing to the lack of specificity of these symptoms. However, they may be of considerable clinical importance because they often appear hours or days before major manifestations of the disease and may mimic a variety of other acute abdominal conditions. The pain is usually epigastric or periumbilical, but may be accompanied by guarding and at times can be virtually indistinguishable from acute appendicitis. Both the temperature and sedimentation rate tends to be higher than in appendicitis, but if the latter cannot be excluded, surgery may be necessary.

New diagnostic techniques for rheumatic carditis
Echocardiography

The use of echocardiography to detect rheumatic carditis is discussed in the following Chapter 4, entitled, *Diagnosis of rheumatic fever and assessment of valvular disease using echocardiography.*

Endomyocardial biopsy

Since myocarditis is an obligatory component of cardiac involvement in RF (8), the value of endomyocardial biopsy has been investigated for diagnosing rheumatic carditis (39). To establish the histological characteristics of carditis, endomyocardial biopsies from patients presenting with a first episode of RF were compared to biopsies from patients with quiescent chronic RHD. The results demonstrated that myocarditis was virtually absent (defined by the Dallas criteria to be focal or diffuse myocytic necrosis associated with cellular infiltration of mononuclear lymphocytes). Instead, there was evidence of interstitial inflammation that ranged from perivascular mononuclear cellular infiltration, to histiocytic aggregates and Aschoff nodule formation. Histiocytic aggregates and Aschoff nodules were identified in only 30% of patients. On the other hand, Aschoff nodules were seen in 40% of the endomyocardial biopsies taken from patients with preexisting RHD and who developed a possible recurrence of rheumatic carditis with CHF. These results suggested that an endomyocardial biopsy is not likely to provide additional diagnostic information for patients with clinical carditis in a primary episode of RF. The results also suggested that an onset of unexplained CHF in patients with established RHD, and who presented with only minor manifestations of RF and elevated antistreptolysin-O titers, would indicate a high probability of rheumatic carditis, and that an invasive test may not be needed for the diagnosis.

Radionuclide imaging

Radionuclide techniques are simple, noninvasive modalities that have been commonly used to evaluate a variety of cardiovascular disorders. The pathology of rheumatic myocarditis is characterized predominantly by the presence of myocardial inflammation, with some damage to myocardial cells (*39, 40*). Gallium-67 (*41*), radiolabelled leukocytes (*42, 43*), and radiolabelled antimyosin antibody (*44*) have all been used to image myocardial inflammation. Although radionuclide imaging has been used successfully to identify rheumatic carditis by non-invasive means, there is not enough experience with such methods to allow them to be used for the routine diagnosis of RF. However, the results of these studies have revealed that gallium-67 imaging has better diagnostic characteristics than antimyosin scintigraphy; and the results also confirmed that rheumatic carditis is predominantly infiltrative, rather than degenerative, in nature.

References

1. **Jones TD.** Diagnosis of rheumatic fever. *Journal of the American Medical association*, 1944, **126**:481–484.

2. **Rutstein DD et al.** Report of the Committee on Standards and Criteria for Programs of Care of the Council of Rheumatic Fever and Congenital Heart Disease of American Heart Association. Jones Criteria (modified) for guidance in the diagnosis of rheumatic fever. *Circulation*, 1956, **13**: 617–620.

3. **Stollerman GH et al.** Report of the ad hoc Committee on Rheumatic Fever and Congenital Heart Disease of American Heart Association: Jones Criteria (Revised) for guidance in the diagnosis of rheumatic fever. *Circulation*, 1965, **32**:664–668.

4. **Shulman ST et al.** Committee on Rheumatic Fever, Endocarditis and Kawasaki Disease of the American Heart Association. Jones Criteria (Revised) for guidance in the diagnosis of rheumatic fever. *Circulation*, 1984, **70**:204A–208A.

5. **Dajani AS et al.** Special writing group of the Committee on Rheumatic fever, Endocarditis and Kawasaki disease of the Council of Cardiovascular disease in the young of the American Heart Association. Guidelines for the diagnosis of rheumatic fever: Jones criteria 1992 Update. *Journal of the American Medical Association*, 1992, **268**:2069–2073.

6. *Rheumatic fever and rheumatic heart disease. Report of a WHO study group*. Geneva, World Health Organization, 1988 (Technical Report Series, No. 764).

7. **Okuni M.** Problems in clinical application of revised Jones diagnostic criteria for rheumatic fever. *Japanese Heart Journal*, 1971, **12**:436–441.

8. **Massell BF, Narula J.** Rheumatic fever and rheumatic carditis. In: Braunwald E, Abelman WH, eds. *The atlas of heart diseases*. Philadelphia, Current Medicine, 1994:10.1–10.20.

9. **Feinstein AR, Stern EK.** Clinical effects of recurrent attacks of acute rheumatic fever: a prospective epidemiologic study of 105 episodes. *Journal of Chronic Diseases*, 1967, **20**:13–27.

10. **Kuttner AG, Meyer FE.** Carditis during second attack of rheumatic fever: its incidence in patients without clinical evidence of cardiac involvement in their initial rheumatic fever episode. *New England Journal of Medicine*, 1963, **268**:1259–1262.

11. **Narula J et al.** Can Antimyosin scintigraphy supplement the Jones Criteria in the diagnosis of active rheumatic carditis? *American Journal of Cardiology*, 1999, **84**:746–750.

12. **Feinstein AR, Spagnuolo M.** Mimetic features of rheumatic fever recurrences. *New England Journal of Medicine*, 1960, **262**:533–540.

13. **Markowitz M.** Evolution and critique of changes in Jones' criteria for diagnosis of acute rheumatic fever. *New Zealand Medical Journal*, 1988, **101**:392–394.

14. **KrishnaKumar R et al.** Epidemiology of streptococcal pharyngitis, rheumatic fever and rheumatic heart disease. In: Narula J et al., eds. *Rheumatic fever*. Washington, DC, American Registry of Pathology, 1999:41–68.

15. **Kaplan EL, Narula J.** Echocardiographic diagnosis of rheumatic fever. *Lancet*, 2001, **358**(9297):2000.

16. **Essop MR, Wisenbaugh T, Sareli P.** Evidence against a myocardial factor as the cause of left ventricular dilation in active rheumatic carditis. *Journal of the American College of Cardiology*, 1993, **22**:826–829.

17. **Edwards BS, Edwards JE.** Congestive heart failure in rheumatic carditis: valvular or myocardial origin. *Journal of the American College of Cardiology*, 1993, **22**:830–831.

18. **Tan AT, Mah PK, Chia BL.** Cardiac tamponade in acute rheumatic carditis. *Annals of the Rheumatic Diseases,* 1983, **42**:699–701.

19. **Feinstein AR et al.** Rheumatic fever in children and adolescents. A long-term epidemiologic study of subsequent prophylaxis, streptococcal infections, and clinical sequelae. VI. Clinical features of streptococcal infection and rheumatic recurrences. *Annals of Internal Medicine*, 1964, **60**(Suppl. 5):68–86.

20. **Sanyal SL et al.** Sequelae of the initial attack of acute rheumatic fever in children from North India: a prospective 5-year follow-up study. *Circulation*, 1982, **65**:375–379.

21. **Svartman M et al.** Immunoglobulins and complement components in synovial fluid of patients with acute rheumatic fever. *The Journal of Clinical Investigation*, 1975, **56**:111–117.

22. **Hubbard WN, Hughes GR.** Streptococci and reactive arthritis. *Annals of the Rheumatic Diseases*, 1982, **41**:435.

23. **Deighton C.** Beta haemolytic streptococci and reactive arthritis in adults. *Annals of the Rheumatic Diseases*, 1993, **52**:475–482.

24. **Schaffer FM et al.** Poststreptococcal reactive arthritis and silent carditis: a case report and review of the literature. *Pediatrics*, 1994, **93**:837–839.

25. **Pinals RS.** Polyarthritis and fever. *New England Journal of Medicine,* 1994, **330**:769–774.

26. **Zvaifler NJ.** Chronic postrheumatic-fever (Jaccoud's) arthritis. *New England Journal of Medicine*, 1962, **267**:10–14.

27. **Bisno A.** Noncardiac manifestations of rheumatic fever. In: Narula et al., eds. *Rheumatic fever.* Washington, DC, American Registry of Pathology, 1994:245–256.

28. **Aron AM, Freeman JM, Carter S.** The natural history of Sydenham's chorea: review of the literature and long-term evaluation with emphasis on cardiac sequelae. *American Journal of Medicine*, 1965, **38**:83–95.

29. **Markowitz M, Gordis L.** *Rheumatic fever*, 2nd ed. Philadelphia, WB Saunders Co., 1972.

30. **Al-Eissa A.** Sydenham's chorea: a new look at an old disease. British Journal of Clinical Practice, 1993, **47**:14–16.

31. **Berrios X et al.** Are all recurrences of "pure" Sydenham's chorea true recurrences of acute rheumatic fever? *Journal of Pediatrics*, 1985, **107**:867–872.

32. **Asherson RA et al.** Chorea in system lupus erythematosus and "lupus-like" disease: association with antiphospholipid antibodies. *Seminars in Arthritis and Rheumatology*, 1987, **16**:253–259.

33. **Sahn DJ, Maciel BC.** Physiological valvular regurgitation: Doppler echocardiography and potential for iatrogenic heart disease. *Circulation,* 1988, **78**:1075–1077.

34. **Tompkins DG et al.** Long term prognosis of rheumatic fever patients receiving regular intramuscular benzathine penicillin. *Circulation*, 1972, 45:543–551.

35. United Kingdom and United States Joint Report on Rheumatic Heart Disease. The natural history of rheumatic fever and rheumatic heart disease. Ten-year report of a cooperative clinical trial of ACTH, cortisone, and aspirin. *Circulation*, 1965, 32:457–476.

36. **Massell BF, Fyler DC, Roy SB.** The clinical picture of rheumatic fever: diagnosis, immediate prognosis, course and therapeutic implications. *American Journal of Cardiology,* 1958, 1:436–439.

37. **Veasy LG, Tani LY, Hill HR.** Persistence of acute rheumatic fever in the intermountain area of the United States. *Journal of Pediatrics*, 1994, 125:673–674.

38. **Al-Eissa YA.** Acute rheumatic fever during childhood in Saudi Arabia. Annals of Tropical Paediatrics, 1991, 11:225–231.

39. **Narula J et al.** Endomyocardial biopsies in acute rheumatic fever. *Circulation*, 1993, 88:2198–2205.

40. **Narula J et al.** Acute myocarditis masquerading as myocardial infarction. *New England Journal of Medicine*, 1993, 328(2):100–104.

41. **Calegaro JU et al.** Galio-67 na febre rheumatica: experiencia preliminary. [Gallium-67 in rheumatic fever: preliminary experience.] *Arquivos Brasileiros de Cardiologia*, [*Brazilian Archives of Cardiology*] 1991, 56:487–492.

42. **Kao CH, Wang SJ, Yeh SH.** Detection of myocarditis in dilated cardiomyopathy by Tc-99m HMPAO WBC myocardial imaging in a child. *Clinical Nuclear Medicine*, 1992, 17:678–679.

43. **Kao CH et al.** Comparison of Tc-99m HMPAO labeled white blood scanning for the detection of carditis in the differentiation of rheumatic fever and inactive rheumatic heart disease in children. *Nuclear Medicine Communications*, 1992, 1:478–481.

44. **Narula J, Chandrashekhar Y, Rahimtoola SH.** Echoes of change: diagnosis of active rheumatic carditis. *Circulation*, 1999, 100:1576–1581.

45. **Markowitz M.** Evolution of the Jones criteria for the diagnosis of acute rheumatic fever. In: Narula J et al., eds. *Rheumatic fever.* Washington, DC, American Registry of Pathology, 1999:299–306.

5. Diagnosis of rheumatic fever and assessment of valvular disease using echocardiography

The advent of echocardiography

Echocardiography is an imaging technique that rapidly evolved and matured, and currently it is a key component in the diagnosis of heart disease. The technique includes transthoracic, transesophageal and intracardiac echocardiography (1–3). Three-dimensional and even four-dimensional echocardiography have also been developed (4). To diagnose rheumatic carditis and assess valvular disease, however, M-mode, two-dimensional (2D), 2D echo-Doppler and colour flow Doppler echocardiography are sufficiently sensitive and provide specific information not previously available. Of these, M-mode echocardiography provides parameters for assessing ventricular function, while 2D echocardiography provides a realistic real-time image of anatomical structure. Two-dimensional echo-Doppler and colour flow Doppler echocardiography are most sensitive for detecting abnormal blood flow and valvular regurgitation.

The use of 2D echo-Doppler and colour flow Doppler echocardiography may prevent the overdiagnosis of a functional murmur as valvular heart disease (5). Similarly, the overinterpretation of physiological or trivial valvular regurgitation may result in a misdiagnosis of iatrogenic valvular disease (6, 7). Accurate interpretation of the echocardiographic signals is therefore important.

Echocardiography and physiological valvular regurgitation

Two-dimensional echo-Doppler and colour flow Doppler echocardiography have permitted all audible valvular regurgitation to be detected, even the physiological, functional, trivial or so-called "normal" flow disturbance that may occur when normal valves close (7–11). Utilizing colour flow Doppler echocardiography, physiological regurgitation is characteristically localized at the region immediately below or above the plane of valve leaflets (or within 1.0 cm), and the signals are short and the maximum regurgitant area small. The appearance of physiological valvular regurgitation in healthy subjects with structurally normal hearts varies with the devices, sensitivity, penetration power and techniques used, with changes in systemic and pulmonary vascular resistance and pressure, and with body habitus and age (3, 6, 7, 9, 12). The prevalence of physiological valvular regurgitation in normal people varied by valve: mitral regurgitation was present in 2.4–45% of normal individuals (7, 9), aortic regurgitation in 0–33% (9, 12), tricuspid regurgitation in 6.3–95% (9, 13), and pulmonary regurgitation in 21.9–92% of normal individuals (9, 12).

The role of echocardiography in the diagnosis of acute rheumatic carditis and in assessing valvular regurgitation

Clinical rheumatic carditis

Echocardiographic images provide information about the size of atria and ventricles, valvular thickening, leaflet prolapse, coaptation failure, restriction of leaflet motility, and ventricular dysfunction (8, 14–18). In 25% of patients with acute rheumatic carditis, focal nodules were found on the bodies and tips of the valve leaflets, but the nodules disappeared on follow-up (17).

Congestive heart failure in patients with rheumatic carditis appears to be invariably associated with severe mitral and/or aortic valve insufficiency (16, 17). Myocardial factor or myocardial dysfunction appeared not to be the main cause of congestive heart failure, as the percent fractional shortening of the left ventricle in such patients with heart failure has been found to be normal, and they improved rapidly after surgery (16, 17, 19). The pathogenesis of severe mitral regurgitation has been found to be owing to a combination of valvulitis, mitral annular dilatation and leaflet prolapse, with or without chordal elongation (16, 17). Chordal rupture occurs in some patients with rheumatic carditis requiring an emergency mitral valve repair (14, 20).

Echo-Doppler and colour flow Doppler imaging may also provide supporting evidence for a diagnosis of rheumatic carditis in patients with equivocal murmur, or with polyarthritis and equivocal minor manifestations (10, 17).

Classification of the severity of valvular regurgitation using echocardiography

Traditionally, the severity of valvular regurgitation has been classified according to a five-point scale (0+, 1+, 2+, 3+ and 4+), based on the echocardiographic findings with angiocardiographic correlations (21–24). But based on colour flow Doppler mapping, it has been suggested that the severity of mitral and aortic valvular regurgitation may be classified into a six-point scale as follows (21–24):

0:   Nil, including physiological or trivial regurgitant jet <1.0 cm, narrow, small, of short duration, early systolic at mitral valve or early diastolic at aortic valve.

0+: Very mild regurgitant jet, more than 1.0 cm, wider, localized immediately above or below the valve, throughout systole at the mitral valve or diastole at the aortic valve (clinically, no murmur audible).

1+: Mild regurgitant jet.

2+: Moderate regurgitant jet, longer and at a wider area.

3+: Moderately severe regurgitant jet, reaching the entire left atrium (mitral regurgitation) or left ventricle (aortic regurgitation).

4+: Severe regurgitant jet, diffusely into the enlarged left atrium, with systolic backward flow into pulmonary veins (mitral valve); markedly enlarged left ventricle filled with regurgitant jets (aortic valve).

Diagnosis of rheumatic carditis of insidious onset

In patients with rheumatic carditis of insidious onset, or indolent carditis, as defined in the 1992 update of the Jones criteria (25), echocardiography serves to establish the diagnosis of mitral and/or aortic insufficiency, after excluding the non-rheumatic causes, such as congenital mitral valve cleft and/or anomalies, degenerative floppy mitral valve, bicuspid aortic valve; and acquired valvular diseases due to infective endocarditis, systemic disease and others. Silent, but significant, very mild (grade 0+) mitral and/or aortic valvular regurgitation may be transient or persistent, even for years (26). It is recommended that such significant mitral and/or aortic regurgitation be labelled as probable rheumatic heart disease (RHD) until proven otherwise, and that the patients have long-term follow-up studies and be placed on secondary rheumatic fever (RF) prophylaxis. In cases of indolent rheumatic carditis, the cardiomegaly and valvular regurgitation may improve, and valve competency may even be restored (26, 27).

The use of echocardiography to assess chronic valvular heart disease

Two-dimensional echocardiography can display the anatomical pathology of the mitral, aortic, tricuspid and (less well) pulmonary valves, and the valvular annulus and apparatus can be delineated. Colour flow Doppler imaging has gained wide acceptance for qualitatively and quantitatively evaluating the flow characteristics across the valve, as well as for evaluating the severity of the flow pathology (11, 22, 28, 29). Congenital, as well as acquired, valvular disease of non-rheumatic origin has to be excluded. Echocardiography may assist physicians to decide the timing of surgical intervention for diseased valves (29).

Diagnosis of recurrent rheumatic carditis

In patients with preexisting RHD, recurrence of RF is almost invariably associated with carditis, manifested as pericarditis; new valvular regurgitation and/or aggravation of the existing valve lesions; increased cardiac enlargement; and congestive heart failure. These findings are easily and accurately detected and displayed by echocardiography.

Diagnosis of subclinical rheumatic carditis

Diagnosis of rheumatic carditis traditionally depends on detecting typical mitral murmurs and/or aortic valvular regurgitation. Two-dimensional echo-Doppler and colour flow Doppler echocardiography can detect silent, but significant, mitral and aortic regurgitation in patients with acute RF (*30–36*). Echocardiographic images reveal: (i) a regurgitant jet >1 cm in length; (ii) a regurgitant jet in at least two planes; (iii) a mosaic colour jet with a peak velocity >2.5 m/s; and (iv) the jet persists throughout systole (mitral valve) and diastole (aortic valve) (*30, 32, 37–40*).

Based on the presence of very mild "silent but significant" valvular regurgitation, a new category of "subclinical carditis", "echocarditis" or "asymptomatic carditis" has been proposed in patients with chorea and polyarthritis (*30–35, 37, 41, 42*). In such cases of subclinical rheumatic carditis, annular dilatation, leaflet prolapse, and elongation of the anterior mitral chordae were observed, indicating that the valve might have been sensitized or damaged (*30, 33*). Patients with subclinical valvular regurgitation may develop an audible murmur in two weeks (*31*), may continue without audible murmur for 18 months to five years (*35–37*), or may progress to irreversible sequelae, such as mitral stenosis (*35*). Although other studies do not support these findings (*10, 43, 44*), 2D echo-Doppler echocardiography detected trivial-to-mild mitral valvular regurgitation in 38–45% of normal/healthy children (*7, 9, 10*), and in even higher proportions of febrile patients (*10*).

These results confirm the usefulness of 2D echo-Doppler and colour flow Doppler echocardiography for diagnosing subclinical rheumatic carditis. However, the use of echocardiography to detect left-side valvular regurgitation and confirm a diagnosis of subclinical rheumatic carditis remains controversial. As such, until the results of long-term encompassing prospective studies are available to substantiate the therapeutic and prognostic importance of subclinical rheumatic carditis, the addition of this criterion to the Jones criteria cannot be justified (*10, 43–47*). However, the acute management of such patients and the duration of secondary prophylaxis would not change significantly, even if a diagnosis of subclinical carditis were made (*10, 43, 44*).

It is also important to recognize that technical expertise with colour flow Doppler echocardiography is necessary to make an accurate diagnosis of subclinical carditis and to avoid overdiagnosis. In developing countries, where the majority of RF cases occur, such expertise and facilities are available in only a limited number of centres. As a result, the impact of erroneous diagnoses of rheumatic carditis based on subclinical echocardiographic findings should not be underestimated, nor should the potentially adverse consequences to patients and health systems in such settings (*10, 44*).

Conclusions: the advantages and disadvantages of Doppler echocardiography

There are significant advantages in using echocardiography to detect valvulitis. Foremost, is its superior sensitivity in detecting rheumatic carditis, which should prevent patients with carditis from being misclassified as noncarditic and placed on abbreviated secondary prophylaxis, in line with the more benign prognosis. It is reasonable to accept that valvular regurgitation may not always be detected by routine clinical auscultation. Even in the Irvington House reports, a number of patients in with no audible murmurs in the first attack of RF developed RHD on follow up (*48, 49*). This suggests that carditis was missed by clinical examination, even in the golden era of clinical auscultation. The likelihood of misclassification is higher now, since clinical auscultatory skills of training physicians are suboptimal, at least in countries where RF is declining (*50, 51*). A second advantage of echocardiography is that it should allow the valve structure to be detected, as well as nonrheumatic causes of valvular dysfunction (e.g. mitral valve prolapse, bicuspid aortic valve), and may prevent patients from being mislabeled as cases of rheumatic carditis.

On the other hand, there are logistical problems with the universal use of echocardiography to detect RF, including the likelihood of detecting carditis in a large proportion of RF patients. This could be ascribed either to the high sensitivity of Doppler echocardiography for diagnosing valvular regurgitation, or to the overdiagnosis of physiological valvular regurgitation as an organic dysfunction, or to both. Another logistical problem with universally applying echocardiography stems from the observation that the use of echo-Doppler echocardiography resulted in a diagnosis of carditis in 90–100% of RF patients. This prevalence of carditis in RF patients is significantly higher than that reported clinically, and the utility of a test that diagnoses a disease characteristic (such as carditis in RF) in almost every patient with RF is questionable.

Finally, in developing countries, which bear the brunt of RF disease, it is unlikely that echocardiographic facilities will be widely available (*52*). Moreover, most of the RF episodes in developing countries are recurrences in patients with established RHD, and the ability of echo-Doppler echocardiography to detect the recurrence of subclinical carditis remains unclear, unless there is an interval change in echo-Doppler findings from a previous echocardiogram. But in many developing countries, it is unreasonable to expect that previous echocardiograms or records will be available for comparison.

References

1. **Feigenbaum H, Zaky A, Waldhausen JA.** Use of ultrasound in the diagnosis of pericardial effusion. *Annals of Internal Medicine*, 1966, **65**:443–452.

2. **Seward JB et al.** Transesophageal echocardiography: technique, anatomic correlations, implementation, and clinical applications. *Mayo Clinic Proceedings*, 1988, **63**:649–680.

3. **Minich LL et al.** Role of echocardiography in the diagnosis and follow-up evaluation of rheumatic carditis. In: Narula et al., eds. *Rheumatic fever.* Washington, DC, American Registry of Pathology, **1994**:307–318.

4. **Sahn DJ.** Directions for the use of intracardiac high-frequency ultrasound scanning for monitoring pediatric interventional catheterization procedures. *Echocardiography*, 1990, **7**:465–468.

5. **Pandian NG et al.** Three-dimensional and four-dimensional transesophageal echocardiographic imaging of the heart and aorta in humans using a computed tomographic imaging probe. *Echocardiography*, 1992, **9**:677–687.

6. **Regmi PR, Pandey MR.** Prevalence of rheumatic fever and rheumatic heart disease in school children of Kathmandu city. *Indian Heart Journal*, 1997, **49**:518–520.

7. **Shah PM.** Quantitative assessment of mitral regurgitation. *Journal of the American College of Cardiology*, 1989, **13**:591–593.

8. **Yoshida K et al.** Colour Doppler evaluation of valvular regurgitation in normal subjects. *Circulation*, 1988, **78**:840–847.

9. **Lembo NJ et al.** Mitral valve prolapse in patients with prior rheumatic fever. *Circulation*, 1988, **77**:830–836.

10. **Brand A, Dollberg S, Keren A.** The prevalence of valvular regurgitation in children with structurally normal hearts: a colour Doppler echocardiographic study. *American Heart Journal*, 1992, **123**:177–180.

11. **Narula J, Chandrasekhar Y, Rohimtoola S.** Diagnosis of acute rheumatic carditis: the echoes of change. *Circulation*, 1999, **100**:1576–1581.

12. **Shah PM.** Quantitative assessment of mitral regurgitation. *Journal of the American College of Cardiology*, 1989, **13**:591–593.

13. **Kostucki W et al.** Pulsed Doppler regurgitant flow patterns of normal valves. *American Journal of Cardiology*, 1986, **58**:309–313.

14. **Yock PG, Schnittger I, Popp RL.** Is continuous wave Doppler too sensitive in diagnosing pathologic valvular regurgitation? *Circulation*, 1984, **70**(II):381.

15. **Marcus RH et al.** Functional anatomy of severe mitral regurgitation in active rheumatic carditis. *American Journal of Cardiology*, 1989, **63**:577–584.

16. **Essop MR, Wisenbaugh T, Sareli P.** Evidence against a myocardial factor as the cause of left ventricular dilation in active rheumatic carditis. *Journal of the American College of Cardiology*, 1993, **22**:826–829.

17. **Vasan RS et al.** Echocardiographic evaluation of patients with acute rheumatic fever and rheumatic carditis. *Circulation*, 1996, **94**:73–82.

18. **Zhou LY, Lu K.** Inflammatory valvular prolapse produced by acute rheumatic carditis: echocardiographic analysis of 66 cases of acute rheumatic carditis. *International Journal of Cardiology*, 1997, **58**:175–178.

19. **Edwards BS, Edwards JE.** Congestive heart failure in rheumatic carditis: valvular or myocardial origin? *Journal of the American College of Cardiology*, 1993, **22**:830–831.

20. **Wu YN et al.** Rupture of chordae tendineae in acute rheumatic carditis: report of one case. *Acta Paediatrica Sinica*, 1992, **33**:376–382.

21. **Helmcke F et al.** Colour Doppler assessment of mitral regurgitation with orthogonal planes. *Circulation*, 1987, **75**:175–183.

22. **Spain MG et al.** Quantitative assessment of mitral regurgitation by Doppler colour flow imaging: angiographic and hemodynamic correlations. *Journal of the American College of Cardiology*, 1989, **13**:585–590.

23. **Wu YT, Chang AC, Chin AJ.** Semiquantitative assessment of mitral regurgitation by Doppler colour flow imaging in patients aged <20 years. *American Journal of Cardiology*, 1993, **71**:727–732.

24. **Nakatani S et al.** Noninvasive estimation of left ventricular end-diastolic pressure using transthoracic Doppler-determined pulmonary venous atrial flow reversal. *American Journal of Cardiology*, 1994, **73**:1017–1018.

25. American Heart Association guidelines for the diagnosis of rheumatic fever: Jones criteria, 1992 update. *Journal of the American Medical Association*, 1992, **268**:2069–2073.

26. **Lue HC et al.** Long-term outcome of patients with rheumatic fever receiving benzathine penicillin G prophylaxis every three weeks versus every four weeks. *Journal of Pediatrics*, 1994, **125**:812–816.

27. **Lue HC et al.** Three-versus four-week administration of benzathine penicillin G: effects on incidence of streptococcal infections and recurrences of rheumatic fever. *Pediatrics*, 1996, **97**:984–988.

28. **Rodriguez L et al.** Validation of the proximal flow convergence method. Calculation of orifice area in patients with mitral stenosis. *Circulation*, 1993, **88**:1157–1165.

29. **Donooan CL, Starling MR.** Role of echocardiography in the timing of surgical intervention for chronic mitral and aortic regurgitation. In: Otto CM, ed. *The practice of clinical echocardiography*. Philadelphia, PA, WB Saunders Co., 1997:327–354.

30. **Folger GM, Hajar R.** Doppler echocardiographic findings of mitral and aortic valvular regurgitation in children manifesting only rheumatic arthritis. *American Journal of Cardiology*, 1989, **63**:1278–1280.

31. **Abernethy M et al.** Doppler echocardiography and the early diagnosis of acute rheumatic fever. *Australian and New Zealand Journal of Medicine*, 1994, **24**:530–535.

32. Wilson NJ, Neutze JM. Echocardiographic diagnosis of subclinical carditis in acute rheumatic fever (editorial). *International Journal of Cardiology*, 1995, **50**:1–6.

33. Agarwal PK et al. Usefulness of echocardiography in detection of subclinical carditis in acute rheumatic polyarthritis and rheumatic chorea. *Journal of the Association of Physicians of India*, 1998, **46**:937–938.

34. Calleja HB, Guzman SV. Advocacy for echocardiography in Jones criteria for the diagnosis of rheumatic fever. In: Calleja HB, Guzman SV, eds. *Rheumatic fever and rheumatic heart disease*. Manila, Philippine Foundation for the Prevention and Control of Rheumatic Fever and Rheumatic Heart Disease, **2001**:27–33.

35. Figueroa FE et al. Prospective comparison of clinical and echocardiographic diagnosis of rheumatic carditis: long term follow up of patients with subclinical disease. *Heart*, 2001, **85**:407–410.

36. Voss LM et al. Intravenous immunoglobulin in acute rheumatic fever: a randomized controlled trial. *Circulation*, 2001, **103**:401–406.

37. Folger GM et al. Occurrence of valvular heart disease in acute rheumatic fever without evident carditis: colour flow Doppler identification. *British Heart Journal*, 1992, **67**:434–438.

38. Zucker N et al. A common colour flow Doppler finding in the mitral regurgitation of acute rheumatic fever. *Echocardiography*, 1991, **8**:627–631.

39. Cotrim C et al. O ecocardiograma no primeiro surto de fibre reumática na crianca. [The echocardiogram in the first attack of rheumatic fever in childhood.] *Revista Portuguesa do Cardiologia, [Portuguese Journal of Cardiology,]* 1994, **13**:581–586.

40. Minich LL et al. Doppler echocardiography distinguishes between physiologic and pathologic "silent" mitral regurgitation in patients with rheumatic fever. *Clinical Cardiology*, 1997, **11**:924–926.

41. Veasy LG, Tani LY, Hill HR. Persistence of acute rheumatic fever in the intermountain area of the United States. *Journal of Pediatrics*, 1994, **124**:9–16.

42. Hilario MO et al. The value of echocardiography in the diagnosis and follow up of rheumatic carditis in children and adolescents: a 2 years prospective study. *Journal of Rheumatology*, 2000, **27**:1082–1086.

43. Vasan RS et al. Echocardiographic evaluation of patients with acute rheumatic fever and rheumatic carditis. *Circulation*, 1996, **94**:73–82.

44. Narula J, Kaplan EL. Echocardiogrphic diagnosis of rheumatic fever. *Lancet*, 2001, **358**(9297):2000.

45. Dajani AS et al. American Heart Association guidelines for the diagnosis of rheumatic fever: Jones criteria, updated 1992. *Circulation*, 87(1):302–307.

46. *Joint WHO/ISFC meeting on RF/RHD control with emphasis on primary prevention. Geneva, 7–9 September 1994*. Geneva, World Health Organization, 1994 (WHO/CVD 94.1).

47. Ferrieri P. AHA scientific statement: proceedings of the Jones Criteria Working Group. *Circulation*, 2002, **106**:2521–2523.

48. **Taranta A et al.** Rheumatic fever in children and adolescents. A long-term epidemiologic study of subsequent prophylaxis, streptococcal infections, and clinical sequelae. V. Relation of the rheumatic fever recurrence rate per streptococcal infection to preexisting clinical features of the patients. *Annals of Internal Medicine*, 1964, **60**(Suppl 5):58–67.

49. **Feinstein AR et al.** Rheumatic fever in children and adolescents. A long-term epidemiologic study of subsequent prophylaxis, streptococcal infections, and clinical sequelae. VI. Clinical features of streptococcal infection and rheumatic recurrences. *Annals of Internal Medicine*, 1964, **60**(Suppl 5):68–86.

50. **Mangione S et al.** The teaching and practice of cardiac auscultation during internal medicine and cardiology training. *Annals of Internal Medicine*, 1993, **119**:47–54.

51. **Shaver JA.** Cardiac auscultation: a cost-effective diagnostic skill. *Current Problems in Cardiology*, 1995, **20**:441–532.

52. **Vijaykumar M et al.** Incidence of rheumatic fever and prevalence of rheumatic heart disease in India. *International Journal of Cardiology*, 1994, **43**:221–228.

6. The role of the microbiology laboratory in the diagnosis of streptococcal infections and rheumatic fever

Group A streptococci commonly cause pharyngitis/tonsillitis that need treatment with antibiotics, and it is important that streptococcal pharyngitis be promptly diagnosed and treated to prevent rheumatic fever (RF), particularly for high-risk populations (1). The microbiology laboratory plays an important role in ensuring that the documentation of group A streptococcal infections is accurate. It does so by using scientific methods both to determine whether group A streptococci (*Streptococcus pyogenes*) are present on swabs from suspected streptococcal throat infections, and to measure streptococcal serum antibody titres for documenting previous infection. An adequate laboratory system is also vital for RF prevention programmes, and the capabilities of microbiology laboratories should extend beyond diagnostic testing, to providing information about the disease and identifying the streptococcal types causing it (1, 2). The conventional methods and procedures for serologically identifying group A streptococcal infections are described elsewhere (3).

Diagnosis of streptococcal infection

Group A streptococci can be subdivided into more than 130 distinct types, based upon a characterization of the M protein of the cell wall, opacity factors antigens produced by the organism, and by molecular sequencing of the *emm* gene that codes for M protein. A less-specific method is to determine the T-antigen pattern, but similar T antigens may be shared by several different M types (4–7). Nevertheless, all group A streptococci produce hemolysis on blood agar, and have an optimum growth temperature in the range 35–37 °C.

The gold standard for detecting *Streptococcus pyogenes* remains a throat swab cultured on blood agar, although it takes 24–48 hours to produce a result, with the consequent delay in starting antibiotic therapy. If possible, throat swabs should be examined for all patients with clinically suspected streptococcal upper respiratory tract infection. The correct procedure for taking a throat swab is to directly observe the tonsillar-pharyngeal area while vigorously swabbing the tonsils or tonsillar crypts and the posterior pharyngeal wall (2, 4, 8–10). If the swabs have to be transported to a laboratory, care should be taken to avoid conditions that are suboptimal for the survival of streptococci, such as high temperatures and swabs that remain moist for long periods (10). On the growth media in commercial swabs, however, beta–haemolytic streptococci can remain viable for up to 48 hours (9). Cultures negative for S. pyogenes after an overnight incubation should be incubated for another 24 hours. S. pyogenes can be presumptively identified using a 0.04 IU bacitracin differential disc on a purity plate (4), although erroneous results will be obtained if the bacitracin discs are placed on primary cultures.

In some countries a number of kits are commercially available for rapidly detecting group A streptococci on throat swabs, either in a "near-patient" situation or in a laboratory. Most of these tests use an immunological method to detect a carbohydrate cell-wall antigen specific to group A streptococci in material from throat swabs, and do not require expert laboratory skills. Detecting the antigen is the most specific method for confirming the presence of group A streptococci and the kits have reported specificities in the range 85–100%, compared with blood agar cultures (8, 11). False-positive results are unusual and therapeutic decisions can be made with confidence. However, different kits can vary in sensitivity from 31–95% and hence they cannot be used to replace standard blood agar cultures, particularly in populations at high risk for RF. In such circumstances, it is recommended that negative kit results should be confirmed by culturing (2, 8). Neither culturing nor rapid testing can reliably distinguish between an acute streptococcal infection, and a streptococcal carrier (12) with a concomitant viral infection (13). Serological examination for streptococcal antibodies (antistreptolysin-O, antideoxyribonuclease B) is not required for cases of uncomplicated streptococcal upper respiratory tract infection, except in specific cases (e.g. diseases of uncertain etiology). Rather, this method is used to establish a diagnosis of a previous streptococcal infection in acute RF patients (4, 7, 8).

Laboratory tests that support a diagnosis of RF

The diagnosis of RF requires evidence of a prior streptococcal infection (see Jones criteria section). If throat swabs are taken from individuals suspected of acute RF there is no certainty that any isolate recovered is the etiology agent triggering the episode of RF or if the patient could be a streptococcal carrier.

Streptococcal serum antibody tests should be undertaken for all suspected cases of acute RF (9), since these provide evidence for antecedent streptococcal infection and fulfil the clinical criteria for a diagnosis of RF. Although a single elevated antibody titre may be useful for documenting a previous streptococcal infection, it is recommended that an additional test be performed 3–4 weeks after the onset of RF. The most commonly performed and commercially available tests are the antistreptolysin-O test, and the antideoxyribonclease B test (*12, 14*). Kits for the antihyaluronidase test are no longer marketed, and an alternative test that uses the simultaneous detection of several antibodies has been reported to be unreliable (*15*).

The blood titres of antistreptolysin-O, antideoxyribonuclease B and other antibodies raised against extracellular antigens of streptococci reach a peak 3–4 weeks after the acute infection, and usually are maintained for 2–3 months before declining (*12*). In most cases of acute RF, when two antibody tests are used, elevated titres will be found in both tests. But about 20% of individuals with a first attack of RF, and most patients with chorea alone, have low antistreptolysin-O titres (*16*). At least one anti-streptococcal antibody titre should be elevated for a diagnosis of acute RF. A serum antibody is judged to be elevated if the titre exceeds the upper limit of the normal titre range for a community, where upper limit is defined as the titre exceeded by no more than 20% of the population. The range of normal values for each test is variable and depends upon the age of the patient, geographical locale and the season of the year (see Table 6.1; *5, 17–19*). The upper limit of normal can be determined by measuring antibody titres in a subset of sera from individuals without a recent streptococcal infection and who belong to the appropriate age group. An antibody standard, or reference serum with a known titre, should be used as a control with each set of antibody determinations.

Table 6.1
Variation in normal antibody titres with age and/or geography

Age group	Country	ULN (test)[a]	Subjects (N)	Reference
Adults (military)	USA	400 (ASO)	600	*16*
2–4 years		120–160 (ASO)	159	*17*
	USA	60–240 (anti-DNase)		
5–9 years		160–240 (ASO)	695	
		320–640 (anti-DNase)		
10–12 years		240–320 (ASO)	277	
		480–640 (anti-DNase)		
2–5 years	New Zealand	141 (ASO)		*18*
		120 (anti-DNase)		
6–10 years		282 (ASO)		
		400 (anti-DNase)	260	
11–14 years		282 (ASO)		
		600 (anti-DNase)		

[a] ASO = antistreptolysin-O test; anti-Dnase = antideoxyribonuclease B test.

Whenever microbiological testing is used, precise guidelines and standards should be followed. This applies to taking throat swabs, transporting swabs to the laboratory, culturing and identifying the microbes, as well as to the procedures used for the antibody test (*1, 2, 8–10*). It is relatively simple to maintain standards by continuing to train laboratory staff (*3*), and this is achievable by most countries.

The role of the microbiology laboratory in RF prevention programmes

The microbiology laboratory plays important roles in RF prevention programmes at several levels (*20, 21*). Both primary and secondary prevention programmes require laboratory support to detect and measure group A streptococci, and to understand the epidemiology of RF in the population. The epidemiology of RF, in particular, cannot be defined using demographic detail alone: it also requires a knowledge of the behaviour and types of streptococci in the population. The microbiology laboratory also contributes to the study and control of actual outbreaks of group A beta-haemolytic streptococci, and allows any suspected outbreaks to be evaluated accurately.

The following three levels of laboratory expertise are recommended, to meet most needs for diagnostic and reference streptococcal services:

- *Peripheral laboratories* handle immediate routine diagnostic tests, such as throat cultures, and also antibody tests. These laboratories should work closely with clinicians. In certain cases, diagnostic testing may be referred to an intermediate laboratory or to a national streptococcal reference laboratory.
- *Intermediate laboratories* are more centralized and should have greater technical skills or instrumentation than peripheral laboratories. They should be able to handle more specimens and carry out more sophisticated testing.
- *National streptococcal reference laboratories.* All countries should be serviced, either nationally or internationally, by such laboratories that can provide reference strains and expert advice on laboratory standards and training, as well as carry out typing (molecular and traditional) of the streptococcal strains. Laboratories should work closely with WHO collaborating centres for reference and research on streptococci (see Appendix 1) or with national reference laboratory to exchange information and to discuss progress in streptococcal microbiology and epidemiology (*20, 21*).

References

1. **Denny F et al.** Prevention of rheumatic fever. Treatment of the preceding streptococcal infection. *Journal of the American Medical Association*, 1950, **143**:151–153.

2. **Dajani A et al.** Treatment of acute streptococcal pharyngitis and prevention of rheumatic fever: a statement for health professionals. *Pediatrics*, 1995, **96**:758–764.

3. *Laboratory Diagnosis of group A streptococcal infections*. Geneva, World Health Organization, 1996.

4. **Johnson DR, Kaplan EL.** A review of the correlation of T-agglutination patterns and M-protein typing and opacity factor production in the identification of group A streptococci. Journal of medical microbiology 1993 May;**38**(5):311–5.

5. **Shet A, Kaplan EL.** Clinical use and interpretation of group A streptococcal antibody tests: a practical approach for the pediatrician or primary care physician. *Pediatric Infectious Disease Journal*, 2002, **21**(5):420–430.

6. **Kaplan EL, Wooton JT, Johnson DR.** Dynamic epidemiology of group A streptococcal serotypes. *Lancet*, 2002, **359**(9323):2115–2116.

7. **Kaplan EL et al.** Dynamic epidemiology of Group A streptococcal serotypes associated with pharingitis. *Lancet*, 2001, **358**:1334–1337.

8. **Bisno AL et al.** Practice guidelines for the diagnosis and management of group A streptococcal pharyngitis. Infectious Diseases Society of America. *Clinical Infectious Diseases*, 2002, **35**(2):113–125.

9. **Kellogg JA.** Suitability of throat culture procedures for detection of group A streptococci and as reference standards for evaluation of streptococcal antigen detection kits. *Journal of Clinical Microbiology*, 1990, **28**: 165–169.

10. **Redys JJ, Hibbard EW, Borman EK.** Improved dry-swab transportation for streptococcal specimens. *Public Health Reports*, 1968, **83**:143–149.

11. **Geber MA et al.** Antigen detection test for streptococcal pharyngitis; evaluation of sensitivity with respect to true infections. *Journal of Pediatrics*, 1986, **108**:654–657.

12. **Ayoub EM.** Streptococcal antibody tests in rheumatic fever. *Clinical Immunology Newsletter*, 1982, **3**:107–111.

13. **Kaplan, EL.** The group A streptococcal upper respiratory tract carrier state: An enigma. *Journal of Pediatrics*, 1980, **97**(3):337–345.

14. **Ayoub EM, Wannamaker LW.** Evaluation of the streptococcal deoxyribonuclease B and diphosphopyridine nucleotidase antibody tests in acute rheumatic fever and acute glomerulonephritis. *Pediatrics*, 1962, **29**:527–538.

15. Evaluation of the streptozyme test for strepococcal antibodies. *Bulletin of the World Health Organization*, 1986, **64**:504.

16. **Wannamaker LW, Ayoub EM.** Antibody titers in acute rheumatic fever. *Circulation*, 1960, **XXI**:598–561.

17. Gray GC et al. Interpreting a single antistreptolysin O test; a comparison of the "upper limit of normal" and likelihood ratio methods. *Journal of Clinical Epidemiology*, 1993, **46**:1181–1185.

18. Kaplan EL, Rothermal CD, Johnson DR. Antistreptolysin O and anti-deoxyribonuclease B titers: Normal values for children ages 2 to 12 in the United States. *Pediatrics*, 1998, **101**:86–88.

19. Dawson KP, Martin DR. Streptococcal involvement in childhood acute glomerulonephritis: a review of 20 cases at admission. *New Zealand Medical Journal*, 1982, **95**(709):373–376.

20. *Rheumatic fever and rheumatic heart disease. Report of a WHO Study Group*. Geneva, World Health Organization, 1988 (WHO Technical Report Series, No. 764).

21. *The WHO Programme on Streptococcal Disease Complex. Report of a consultation, Geneva, 16–19 February, 1998*. Geneva, World Health Organization (unpublished document EMC/BAC/98.7).

Appendix 1
WHO collaborating centres for reference and research on streptococci (*21*)

— Department of Paediatric, University of Minnesota Medical School, Minneapolis, Minnesota 55455, USA.
— Streptococcus & Diphtheria Reference Unit, Respiratory & Systemic Infection Laboratory, Central Public Health Laboratory, London NW9 5HT, UK.
— Laboratoire de Bactériologie et Mycologie Médicale, Institut Supérieur de la Santé, Ministère de la Santé, I-00144 Roma, Italy.
— National Institute of Public Health, Centre of Epidemiology and Microbiology 100 42 Prague 10, Czech Republic.
— Department of Molecular Microbiology, Research Institute of Experimental Science, St. Petersburg, Russian Federation.

Chronic rheumatic heart disease

It is important to emphasize that medical management of chronic rheumatic heart disease (RHD) must defer to operative intervention when clinical or echocardiographic criteria are met, and when surgery is both accessible and feasible. In many cases, the development of heart failure, particularly when attributable to left ventricular systolic dysfunction, implies that surgery has been inappropriately delayed.

Mitral stenosis

The natural history of mitral stenosis varies across geographical areas. In North America, for example, it is most commonly an indolent and slowly progressive disease, with a latency period as long as 20–40 years between the initial infection and the onset of clinical symptoms (*1, 2*). In developing countries, on the other hand, mitral stenosis progresses much more rapidly, perhaps because of more severe or repeated streptococcal infections, genetic influences, or economic conditions, and may lead to symptoms in the late teens and early twenties (*3*). Survival is >80% at 10 years for untreated patients who are asymptomatic or minimally symptomatic (New York Heart Association (NYHA) Functional Class I/II) at time of diagnosis; 60% of such patients may not experience any progression of symptoms over this time frame (*4*). Once limiting symptoms (Functional Class III/IV) develop, however, survival without intervention predictably worsens and has been estimated at 0–15% over the ensuing 10 years (*4, 5*). Mean survival time falls to less than three years if severe pulmonary hypertension has intervened (*6*). The mortality of untreated patients with mitral stenosis is attributable to progressive heart failure in 60–70% of patients, systemic embolism in 20–30%, pulmonary embolism in 10%, and infection in 1–5% (*7, 8*).

The development of symptoms in patients with mitral stenosis is attributable to either a critical increase in transmitral flow, or a decrease in the diastolic filling period, either or both of which can lead to an increase in left atrial and pulmonary venous pressures and the expression of dyspnea. The initial presentation of patients with even mild-to-moderate mitral stenosis (mitral valve area 1.5–2.0 cm^2) may be precipitated by exercise, emotional upset, fever, pregnancy, or atrial fibrillation, especially with a rapid ventricular response. During the late stages of mitral stenosis, as pulmonary vascular resistance rises and cardiac output falls, fatigue or effort intolerance may play a dominant role. Alternatively, patients may "adapt" to the haemodynamic impairment and inadvertently curtail their activities to the extent that symptoms are minimized despite progressive disease. Severe mitral stenosis is usually defined by a mitral valve area of $\leq1.0\,\mathrm{cm}^2$ (*9*).

There is no medical therapy available to reverse the mechanical obstruction to mitral inflow. Because the left ventricle is protected from any volume or pressure load, there is no indication for empirical treatment in the asymptomatic patient with mild-to-moderate mitral stenosis and normal sinus rhythm. Symptoms of congestion can be treated with diuretics and salt restriction, though care is needed to avoid a critical fall in filling pressures, to the extent that cardiac output and peripheral perfusion suffer. The intermittent use of diuretics may suffice. Digoxin is of no proven benefit in patients with normal sinus rhythm and preserved left ventricular systolic function. Beta-blockers and rate-slowing calcium channel antagonists may be of benefit in some patients by slowing the heart response to exercise. The treatment of haemoptysis must be directed at the root cause, which can vary from pulmonary edema to bronchitis; measures to reduce left atrial and pulmonary venous pressures may be appropriate. Patients with severe stenosis or symptoms of such should be advised against strenuous physical activities (*9*).

Patients with mitral stenosis are particularly susceptible to the development of atrial fibrillation (AF), because of left atrial dilatation in response to valve obstruction, and because of the inflammatory and fibrotic changes caused by the rheumatic process (*10, 11*). Although episodic and paroxysmal at first, AF tends to become persistent over time. With the onset of AF, there is an abrupt loss of the atrial contribution to ventricular filling and as much as a 30% reduction in cardiac output. Under such conditions, there is the potential for a sudden increase in left atrial pressure, especially with rapid ventricular rates due to a critical decrease in diastolic filling times, and the potential for a significant increase in the associated risk of thromboembolism. AF is more common among older patients and, in some studies, has been related to the severity of the stenosis and to the left atrial pressure (*10*).

Among the acquired heart valve lesions, mitral stenosis is associated with the highest risk of systemic thromboembolism. The incidence of systemic embolization, including stroke, among patients with rheumatic mitral valve disease has been estimated at 1.5–4.7% per year. This incidence increases markedly following the onset of AF, and is considerably higher for patients with mitral stenosis, rather than isolated mitral regurgitation (*12*). Patients who suffer a first embolus are at increased risk for a second, particularly within the next six months. Despite claims to the contrary, there are no prospective data to support the contention that successful valvuloplasty (surgical or balloon) obviates the need for long-term anticoagulation therapy in patients who have had an embolus (9). Observational studies have reported significant reductions in the incidence of recurrent emboli among patients treated long-term with warfarin anticoagulation, from rates of approximately 5% per year in untreated patients, to 0.7–0.8% per year in those receiving warfarin (13, 14). In addition, evidence to support the efficacy of anticoagulation for preventing thromboembolism in mitral valve disease can be extrapolated from four large, randomized prospective trials in patients with nonvalvular AF (15–18). In each of these studies, the patients who benefited most from anticoagulant treatment were those at highest risk for embolic events. Patients with mitral stenosis at highest risk for embolic events are those with paroxysmal or persistent AF, or a history of prior embolus. Accordingly, warfarin anticoagulation to an international normalized ratio (INR) of 2.0–3.0 is recommended for these patients. If embolization occurs despite such treatment, an INR of 2.5–3.5 and/or the addition of low dose aspirin (75–100 mg per day) is recommended (9, 19).

The management of AF must be tailored to the clinical context in which it occurs. In all instances, a precipitating cause (fever, anemia, thyrotoxicosis) should be identified and treated. Slowing the ventricular response and providing a diuretic can often restore clinical stability. Agents useful for slowing the ventricular response include beta-blockers, the non-dihydropyridine calcium channel antagonists (diltiazem, verapamil), and digoxin. Beta-blockers and diuretics can be used in pregnant women with little risk to the fetus. With new onset AF of no more than 24–48 hours duration, particularly when rapid and accompanied by symptoms, consideration should be given to direct current cardioversion (when available) to restore sinus rhythm quickly. For AF of more than 48 hours, or of uncertain duration, one of two strategies is recommended, assuming anticoagulation can be administered and monitored, and echocardiography is available (9, 20, 21). The strategies are: (i) control the ventricular rate and use warfarin anticoagulation targeted to a therapeutic INR for three weeks, followed by direct current cardioversion; and (ii) control the ventricular rate, use intravenous unfractionated heparin, trans-oesophageal echocardiography to exclude left atrial thrombus, and direct current cardioversion if negative. If a left atrial thrombus is identified, patients should receive at least three weeks of therapeutic warfarin anticoagulation and undergo repeat trans-oesophageal echocardiography before cardioversion. With either of these two strategies, warfarin anticoagulation is recommended indefinitely thereafter (when feasible), as would also be the case for any patient with a history of prior embolization independent of rhythm. If indefinite anticoagulation is not feasible, a 3–4 week post-cardioversion course is advised (when feasible) to decrease the incidence of embolization during the delayed recovery of the left atrial mechanical function. Although individual exceptions do occur, the success rate of cardioversion falls significantly as a function of left atrial size and the length of time in AF. The empirical use of warfarin as prophylaxis against a first embolus in patients with moderate or severe mitral stenosis, left atrial enlargement (>5.5 cm), and sinus rhythm, is controversial (22).

There are several anti-arrhythmic agents available for the maintenance of sinus rhythm in patients with frequent paroxysms of AF. These are usually given prior to a second or third cardioversion, but their efficacy in patients with mitral valve disease, as measured by their ability both to restore and maintain sinus rhythm, can be difficult to predict given the structural changes in left atrial architecture that underlie the AF. The choice of an individual agent, usually from among the Vaughan-Williams classes IA (quinidine, procainamide, disopyramide), IC (flecainide, propafenone), or III (amiodarone, sotalol), is dictated by the relative safety profile for any given patient, drug-drug interactions, and physician familiarity. These drugs are not readily available in many areas and their electrophysiological effects can be very difficult to monitor. Use of the class IA and class IC agents, for example, may often necessitate the concomitant use of an atrioventricular nodal blocking agent.

At specialized centres, several nonpharmacological interventions have been employed for the treatment of AF, including catheter-delivered radio-frequency ablation, dual-site atrial pacing, atrial cardioverters/defibrillators, and the surgical (Cox) maze procedure (23).

The late stages of uncorrected, severe mitral stenosis may be complicated by the development of pulmonary hypertension, and by failure of the right side of the heart, with edema and ascites. Tricuspid regurgitation commonly co-exists and is more often secondary to right ventricular dilatation, than to primary rheumatic involvement. At this stage, AF is invariably present and the risk of venous thromboembolic disease is greatly increased. Treatment is directed at optimization of fluid status with diuretics and salt/fluid restriction, rate control of AF, anticoagulation, and inotropic support of right ventricular function (if needed). Digoxin is the preferred agent to control ventricular rate; beta-blockers and rate-slowing calcium channel antagonists have negative inotropic effects that could be deleterious in this setting. Nutritional efforts to protect against hypoalbuminemia and the use of graduated compression stockings are also helpful.

Mitral regurgitation

The volume load of chronic mitral regurgitation can be well tolerated for several years. Indeed, the favourable loading conditions may obscure the recognition of left ventricular contractile dysfunction until relatively late in the natural history. Symptoms and/or signs of left ventricular systolic dysfunction (defined by an ejection fraction <0.60, or an end-systolic dimension ≥4.5 cm) are indications for surgery (9). The long-term results of mitral valve surgery are influenced by age, the severity of symptoms, coexistent coronary artery disease, preoperative left ventricular function, the type of surgery (repair vs. replacement), and the presence of AF (9). The onset of symptoms may correlate with the development of AF. Compared with patients with predominant stenosis, patients with isolated mitral regurgitation are less susceptible to thromboembolism with AF, but are more prone to infective endocarditis (10, 24).

A few small-scale studies have suggested that patients with rheumatic (fixed orifice) mitral regurgitation might actually experience haemodynamic worsening following exposure to vasodilators (25–27). These agents, particularly angiotensin converting enzyme inhibitors, are certainly indicated for the treatment of coexistent systemic hypertension or established left ventricular systolic dysfunction, whether or not symptoms are present. Beta-blockers (metoprolol, bisoprolol, carvedilol) and digoxin can be used to manage chronic heart failure owing to left ventricular systolic dysfunction, as currently recommended by consensus guidelines (28). Diuretics should be employed to treat pulmonary or systemic venous congestion. A single trial has suggested that spironolactone may provide additional benefit to NYHA Class III/IV patients, but only a minority of the study participants were receiving beta-blockers and the applicability of these findings to patients with chronic valvular heart disease is uncertain (29).

Atrial fibrillation is managed according to the principles enumerated above for mitral stenosis. In chronic, severe mitral regurgitation, the left atrium can dilate to massive proportions ("giant" left atrium), thus hindering the chances for successful restoration and maintenance of sinus rhythm. Warfarin anticoagulation is recommended when feasible. Pulmonary hypertension and failure of the right side of the heart can occur, but are usually less prominent features of the natural history of mitral regurgitation than they are with mitral stenosis.

Mixed mitral stenosis/regurgitation

Many patients with rheumatic mitral valve disease have important stenotic and regurgitant components owing to commissural fusion and the "fish mouth" deformity imparted by the pathological process. One lesion may predominate, or the components may be more closely balanced, creating a hybrid natural history. Treatment must respect the inherent risks of AF and thromboembolism with mitral stenosis, as well as the chronic left ventricular volume overload of mitral regurgitation. The combined use of diuretics and vasodilators in symptomatic patients may prove challenging, given the more difficult-to-predict effects on filling pressures and systemic perfusion, although the former agents are well tolerated in patients with pulmonary congestion. The indications for anticoagulation, cardioversion, or rate control of AF are the same as would pertain for either lesion in isolation.

Aortic stenosis

The well-known natural history of aortic stenosis has long dictated that surgery be undertaken once symptoms appear. Indeed, survival without valve replacement after the onset of angina, syncope, or heart failure is generally measured at five, three, and two years, respectively (30). For patients with severe aortic stenosis (valve area ≤1.0 cm^2) who develop heart failure and who are not candidates for surgery, diuretics can be provided to alleviate congestion, but special care must be taken to avoid a critical fall in left ventricular preload. Once left ventricular systolic dysfunction intervenes, digoxin can be added; beta-blockers and other drugs with negative inotropic effects should be avoided. Angiotensin converting enzyme inhibitors must also be given with great care in this setting, but may on occasion be helpful in controlling or ameliorating symptoms. AF is an uncommon complication of isolated aortic stenosis, but the associated fall in cardiac output from loss of atrial pump function can be quite deleterious and prompt cardioversion may be necessary. Patients with heart failure and aortic stenosis with "low gradient/low output" should undergo referral and additional testing to determine if the depressed left ventricular function is due to severe, uncorrected aortic stenosis (afterload mismatch) or to a primary cardiomyopathy (31).

Asymptomatic patients with aortic stenosis may require treatment for other, acquired cardiovascular diseases, such as hypertension and coronary artery disease. In the presence of normal left ventricular systolic function, standard doses of angiotensin converting enzyme inhibitors, beta-blockers, and long-acting nitrate preparations are usually well tolerated, though caution is always advised when instituting these medications. Low starting doses are recommended. Several recent studies in patients with degenerative, calcific aortic stenosis have identified smoking, hyperlipidaemia, elevated creatinine, and hypocalcaemia as risk factors for the progression of disease (32–34). Aggressive prevention strategies would seem appropriate for patients with rheumatic disease as well, if only to reduce the incidence of coronary heart disease events, although specific data are lacking. Physical activity need not be restricted in patients with mild aortic stenosis (valve area >1.5 cm²). Patients with moderate aortic stenosis (valve area 1.0–1.5 cm²) should be advised to avoid strenuous activity and competitive sports. Severe aortic stenosis usually mandates a reduction in physical activities to low levels (9).

Aortic regurgitation

Patients with chronic, severe aortic regurgitation usually enjoy a long, yet variable compensated phase characterized by an increase in left ventricular end-diastolic volume, an increase in chamber compliance, and a combination of both eccentric and concentric hypertrophy. Preload reserve is maintained, ejection performance remains normal, and the enormous increase in stroke volume allows preservation of forward output (9). In contrast to the haemodynamic state associated with mitral regurgitation, however, left ventricular afterload progressively increases. Aortic regurgitation thus leads both to volume and pressure overload (9, 24). Vasodilators can favorably alter these loading conditions and may extend the compensated phase of aortic regurgitation prior to the development of symptoms or left ventricular systolic dysfunction (defined as a subnormal resting ejection fraction) that would prompt valve replacement. Preoperative left ventricular function is the most important predictor of postoperative survival.

The natural history of asymptomatic patients with normal systolic function has been well characterized. The rate of progression to symptoms and/or systolic dysfunction has been estimated at less than 6% per year. Thus, these patients can be safely and expectantly followed. Asymptomatic patients with left ventricular dysfunction, however, develop symptoms (angina, heart failure) at a rate of >25% per year, and symptomatic patients with severe aortic regurgitation have an expected mortality that exceeds 10% per year (9). Clinical and noninvasive variables associated with poor outcomes include age, the coexistence of coronary artery disease, the severity of symptoms, resting ejection fraction, end-systolic dimension, end-diastolic dimension, and AF. Asymptomatic patients with normal left ventricular systolic function should avoid isometric exercises, but can otherwise pursue all forms of physical activities including, in some instances, competitive sports. Symptoms or left ventricular dysfunction should prompt a limitation of activities.

Vasodilating agents are recommended for the treatment of patients with severe (3–4+/4+) aortic regurgitation under one of three circumstances (9): (i) short-term administration in preparation for aortic valve replacement in patients with severe heart failure symptoms, or significant left ventricular systolic dysfunction; (ii) long-term administration in patients with symptoms or left ventricular systolic dysfunction who are not considered candidates for valve replacement surgery because of medical comorbidities or patient preference; (iii) long-term administration in asymptomatic patients with normal left ventricular systolic function to extend the compensated phase of aortic regurgitation prior to the need for valve replacement surgery. Vasodilator therapy is generally not recommended for asymptomatic patients with mild-to-moderate aortic regurgitation unless systemic hypertension is also present, as these patients generally do well for years without medical intervention. The goal of long-term therapy in appropriate candidates is to reduce the systolic pressure (afterload), though it is usually difficult to achieve low-to-normal values owing to the augmented stroke volume and preserved contractile function at this stage.

Several small studies have demonstrated haemodynamically beneficial effects with a variety of vasodilators, including nitroprusside, hydralazine, nifedipine, enalapril and quinapril (27). These agents generally reduce left ventricular volumes and regurgitant fraction, with or without a concomitant increase in ejection fraction. Only one study, which compared long-acting nifedipine (60 mg bid) with digoxin in 143 patients followed for six years, has demonstrated that vasodilator therapy can favorably influence the natural history of asymptomatic severe aortic regurgitation (35). The use of nifedipine in this study was associated with a reduction in the need for aortic valve surgery from 34% to 15% over six years. Whether angiotensin converting enzyme inhibitors can provide similar long-term effects has not been conclusively demonstrated in large numbers of patients. Finally, it is important to note that vasodilator therapy is not a substitute for surgery once symptoms and/or left ventricular systolic function intervene, unless there are independent reasons not to pursue aortic valve replacement. Diuretics are recommended to relieve symptoms of pulmonary congestion (dyspnea, orthopnea). Extrapolating from studies of patients with dilated cardiomyopathy, digoxin and spironolactone may be of symptomatic and survival benefit when added to diuretics and angiotensin converting enzyme inhibitors, although data from prospective studies in patients with valvular heart disease are lacking. As noted previously for patients with acute severe aortic regurgitation, beta-blockers, which can slow the heart rate and thus allow greater time for diastolic regurgitation, are contra-indicated. The loss of the atrial contribution to ventricular filling with the onset of fibrillation, as well as a rapid ventricular rate, can result in sudden and significant haemodynamic deterioration. Cardioversion is advised whenever feasible, with the same caveats regarding anticoagulation for thromboembolic prophylaxis, as reviewed above.

Mixed aortic stenosis/regurgitation

Management of patients with mixed aortic valve disease can be quite challenging and depends, in part, on the dominant lesion. Clinical assessment requires integration of both physical examination and echocardiographic data. Symptoms may develop and indications for surgery may be met before the traditional anatomic (valve area) and haemodynamic (ejection fraction) thresholds are reached. The nondominant lesion may exacerbate the pathophysiology imposed by the dominant lesion. Diuretic and/or vasodilator therapies may alter loading conditions in favorable or unfavorable ways, though the former is usually well tolerated in patients with pulmonary congestion. Beta-blockers should be avoided; digoxin may be of benefit once left ventricular systolic function has declined, though its use remains largely empirical.

Multivalvular heart disease

In many patients with chronic RHD both the mitral and aortic valves may be involved, often with mixed lesions in one or both locations. In general, management should be predicated on the identification of the dominant valve lesion and location, though it is recognized that the proximal valve lesion(s) may mask the presence and significance of the more distal valve lesion(s). Thus, the signs of left ventricular volume overload with aortic regurgitation may be attenuated by the presence of significant mitral stenosis, as obstruction to left ventricular inflow restricts filling. Other common combinations include mitral stenosis with tricuspid regurgitation (usually secondary to pulmonary hypertension and right ventricular dilatation), and aortic stenosis with mitral regurgitation. Intermittent or chronic diuretic use to treat symptoms of pulmonary or systemic venous congestion is usually well tolerated. The use of vasodilators must be individualized and depends on the dominant valve lesion, as well as on the expected contribution of the nondominant lesion(s). As is true for the individual lesions, the onset of AF is typically a signal event in the natural history of multivalve disease, is often a clue to the coexistence of mitral involvement in patients followed for aortic disease, and mandates anticoagulation, cardioversion, or rate control as discussed previously.

References

1. **Rowe JC, Bland EF, Sprague HB.** The course of mitral stenosis without surgery: ten and twenty year perspectives. *Annals of Internal Medicine*, 1960, **52**:741–749.

2. **Carroll JD, Feldman T.** Percutaneous mitral balloon valvotomy and the new demographics of mitral stenosis. *Journal of the American Medical Association*, 1993, **270**:1731–1736.

3. **Joswig BC et al.** Contrasting progression of mitral stenosis in Malayans versus American-born Caucasians. *American Heart Journal*, 1982, **104**:1400.

4. **Selzer A, Cohn KE.** Natural history of mitral stenosis: a review. *Circulation*, 1972, **45**:878–890.

5. **Munoz S et al.** Influence of surgery on the natural history of rheumatic mitral and aortic valve disease. *American Journal of Cardiology*, 1975, **35**:234–242.

6. **Ward C, Hancock BW.** Extreme pulmonary hypertension caused by mitral valve disease: natural history and results of surgery. *British Heart Journal*, 1975, **37**:74–78.

7. **Olesen KH.** The natural history of 271 patients with mitral stenosis under medical treatment. *British Heart Journal*, 1962, **24**:349–357.

8. **Roberts WC, Perloff JK.** Mitral valvular disease: a clinicopathologic survey of the conditions causing the mitral valve to function abnormally. *Annals of Internal Medicine*, 1972, **77**:939–975.

9. **Bonow RO et al.** ACC/AHA guidelines for the management of patients with valvular heart disease. *Journal of the American College of Cardiologists*, 1998, **32**:1486–1588.

10. **Moreyra AE et al.** Factors associated with atrial fibrillation in patients with mitral stenosis. A cardiac catheterization study. *American Heart Journal*, 1998, **135**:138–145.

11. **Keren G et al.** Atrial fibrillation and atrial enlargement in patients with mitral stenosis. *American Heart Journal*, 1987, **114**:1146.

12. **Dervall PB et al.** Incidence of stenosis embolism before and after mitral valvotomy. *Thorax*, 1968, **23**:530–540.

13. **Fleming HA, Bailey SM.** Mitral valve disease, systemic embolism, and anticoagulants. *Postgraduate Medical Journal*, 1971, **47**:599–604.

14. **Roy D et al.** Usefulness of anticoagulant therapy in the prevention of embolic complications of atrial fibrillation. *American Heart Journal*, 1986, **112**:1039–1043.

15. **Peterson P et al.** Placebo controlled, randomized trial of warfarin and aspirin for prevention of thromboembolic complications in chronic atrial fibrillation. *Lancet*, 1989, **8631**:175–179.

16. Stroke Prevention in Atrial Fibrillation Study Group Investigators. Preliminary report of the stroke prevention in atrial fibrillation study. *New England Journal of Medicine*, 1990, **322**(12):863–868.

17. The Boston Area Anticoagulation Trial for Atrial Fibrillation Investigators. The effect of low dose warfarin on the risk of stroke in patients with non-rheumatic atrial fibrillation. *New England Journal of Medicine*, 1990, **323**:1505–1511.

18. Ezekowitz MD et al. Warfarin in the prevention of stroke associated with nonrheumatic atrial fibrillation. *New England Journal of Medicine*, 1992, **327**(20):1406–1412.

19. Salem DN et al. Antithrombotic therapy in valvular heart disease. *Chest*, 2001, **119**(Suppl): 207S–219S.

20. Manning WJ et al. Transesophageal echocardiographically facilitated early cardioversion from atrial fibrillation using short term anticoagulation: final results of a prospective 4.5 year study. *Journal of the American College of Cardiologists*, 1995, **25**:1354–1361.

21. Klein AL et al. Use of transesophageal echocardiography to guide cardioversion in patients with atrial fibrillation. *New England Journal of Medicine*, 2001, **344**:1411–1420.

22. Pumphrey CW, Fuster V, Cheseboro HJ. Systemic thromboembolism in valvular heart disease and prosthetic heart valves. *Modern Concepts in Cardiovascular Disease*, 1982, **51**:131–136.

23. Fuster V et al. ACC/AHA/ESC guidelines for the management of patients with atrial fibrillation. *Journal of the American College of Cardiologists*, 2001, **38**:1266.

24. Braunwald E. Valvular heart disease. In: Braunwald E, Zipes D, Libby P, eds. *Heart Disease*, 6th ed. New York, WB Saunders, **2001**: 1643–1713.

25. Weisenbaugh T et al. Effects of a single oral dose of captopril on left ventricular performance in severe mitral regurgitation. *American Journal of Cardiology*, 1992, **69**:348–353.

26. Rothlisberger C, Sareli P, Weisenbaugh T. Comparison of single dose nifedipine and captopril for chronic severe mitral regurgitation. *American Journal of Cardiology*, 1994, **73**:978–981.

27. Levine H, Gaasch W. Vasoactive drugs in chronic regurgitant lesions of the mitral and aortic valves. *Journal of the American College of Cardiologists*, 1996, **28**:1083–1091.

28. Hunt SA et al. ACC/AHA guidelines for the evaluation and management of heart failure in the adult. *Circulation*, 2001, **104**(24): 2998–3007.

29. Pitt B et al. The effect of spironolactone on morbidity and mortality in patients with severe heart failure. *New England Journal of Medicine*, 1999, **341**:709–717.

30. Ross J Jr, Braunwald E. Aortic stenosis. *Circulation*, 1968, **38**:61–67.

31. Carabello B. Aortic stenosis. *New England Journal of Medicine*, 2002, **346**:677–682.

32. **Otto CM et al.** Association of aortic valve sclerosis mortality and morbidity in the elderly. *New England Journal of Medicine*, 1999, **341**:142.

33. **Wilmshurst PT et al.** A case control investigation of the relationship between hyperlipidemia and aortic valve stenosis. *Heart*, 1997, **78**:475.

34. **Stewart BF et al.** Clinical factors associated with calcific aortic valve disease. *Journal of the American College of Cardiologists*, 1997, **29**:630.

35. **Sconamiglio R et al.** Nifedipine in asymptomatic patients with severe aortic regurgitation and normal left ventricular function. *New England Journal of Medicine*, 1994, **331**:689–694.

Pregnancy in patients with rheumatic heart disease

The haemodynamic changes that occur during pregnancy present a challenge to the cardiovascular system in women with RHD and may threaten the well-being and survival of the patient and fetus. The changes can worsen prior haemodynamic alterations and this situation poses a special therapeutic problem. The relevant haemodynamic changes are an increasing heart rate, instability in arterial blood pressure and in systemic and pulmonary resistance, and increased cardiac output. During labour, delivery and the post-partum, these haemodynamic alterations suffer sudden and severe changes that can cause life-threatening complication in these patients. Sometimes, subclinical RHD becomes apparent for the first time during pregnancy (*1–3*).

The management of RHD patients depends on the type and severity of valvular disease. To make a timely decision on the optimal treatment for such patients, it is mandatory that the haemodynamic status of the patient be evaluated, and follow-up evaluations be carried out. These include:

- Following general recommendations that apply to all pregnant RHD patients, including restricting physical activity and salt intake; administering appropriate secondary prophylaxis and avoiding intercurrent infectious diseases; monitoring haemodynamics (mainly for the symptomatic patients).
- Following the status of patients with mitral regurgitation, aortic regurgitation and mild-to-moderate mitral stenosis (NYHA Functional classification Class I and II) and giving medical care as necessary. Patients can be supported with diuretics, digoxin and others, as needed. Angiotensin-converting enzyme inhibitors should not be used during pregnancy.
- Giving special attention to patients with: moderate-to-severe RHD (NYHA Class III and IV, symptomatic heart failure, left ventricular dysfunction, or pulmonary hypertension); mainly mitral stenosis; aortic stenosis; plurivalvular disease and AF; prosthetic heart

valves; and to those under anticoagulant therapy. These patients are at high risk of life-threatening complications during pregnancy and delivery, and in most cases physicians should advise that pregnancy be avoided. However, given the advances in cardiovascular diagnostic and therapeutic techniques, including percutaneous balloon mitral valvotomy and surgical commissurotomy performed during pregnancy, pregnancy could be allowed if the appropriate facilities arc available (*1–9*).

- Warfarin is contraindicated during pregnancy because of teratogenic effects on the foetus.

References

1. Salazar E. Pregnancy in patients with rheumatic cardiopathy. *Archivos Cardiologia de Mexico, [Mexican Archives of Cardiology,]* 2001, 71:S160–S163.

2. Calleja HB, Guzman SV. Pregnancy and rheumatic valvular heart disease. In: Calleja HB, Guzman SV, eds. *Rheumatic fever and rheumatic heart disease: epidemiology, clinical aspects, management and prevention*, 1st ed. Pasig City, Philippines, Medicomm Pacific Inc., **2001**:323–332.

3. Braunwald E. *Heart disease. A textbook of cardiovascular medicine*, 4th ed. Philadelphia, USA, WB Saunders Company, **1992**:1796–1797.

4. Siu SC, Colman JM. Heart disease and pregnancy. *Heart*, 2001, 85:710–715.

5. Barbosa PJ et al. Prognostic factors of rheumatic mitral stenosis during pregnancy and puerperium. *Arqivos Brasileiros de Cardiologia, [Brazilian Archives of Cardiology,]* 2000, **75**(3):215–224.

6. Lin J, Lin Q, Hong S. Retrospective analysis of 266 cases of pregnancy complicated by heart disease. *Zhonghua Fu Chan Ke Za Zhi*, 2000, **35**(6):338–341.

7. de Andrade J et al. The role of mitral valve balloon valvuloplasty in the treatment of rheumatic mitral valve stenosis during pregnancy. *Revista Española de Cardiologia, [Spanish Journal of Cardiology,]* 2001, **54**(5):573–579.

8. Sadler L et al. Pregnancy outcomes and cardiac complications in women with mechanical, bioprosthetic and homograft valves. *British Journal of Obstetrics and Gynaecology*, 2000, **107**(2):245–253.

9. Gupta A et al. Balloon mitral valvotomy in pregnancy: maternal and fetal outcomes. *Journal of the American College of Surgeons*, 1998, **187**(4):409–415.

8. Medical management of rheumatic fever

General measures

Hospital admission may be helpful for confirming a diagnosis of rheumatic fever (RF), for instituting treatment and for educating the patients and family. Initial tests should include a throat culture (or in some circunstances rapid streptococcal detection test), a measurement of streptococcal antibody titres (eg ASO or anti DNase B), an assessment of acute-phase reactants (eg ESR or CRP), a chest X-ray, an electrocardiogram, and an echocardiogram (if facilities are available). A blood culture may help to exclude infective endocarditis (1).

All patients with acute RF should be placed on bed–chair rest and monitored closely for the onset of carditis. In patients with carditis, a rest period of at least four weeks is recommended (2), although physicians should make this decision on an individual basis. Ambulatory restrictions may be relaxed when there is no carditis and when arthritis has subsided (1). Patients with chorea must be placed in a protective environment so they do not injure themselves.

Antimicrobial therapy

Eradication of the pharyngeal streptococcal infection is mandatory to avoid chronic repetitive exposure to streptococcal antigens (2). Ideally, two throat cultures should be performed before starting antibiotics. However, antibiotic therapy is warranted even if the throat cultures are negative. Antibiotic therapy does not alter the course, frequency and severity of cardiac involvement (3). The eradication of pharyngeal streptococci should be followed by long-term secondary prophylaxis to guard against recurrent pharyngeal streptococcal infections.

Suppression of the inflammatory process

It is advisable to avoid premature administration of salicylates or corticosteroids until the diagnosis of RF is confirmed. Aspirin, 100 mg/kg-day divided into 4–5 doses, is the first line of therapy and is generally adequate for achieving a clinical response. In children, the dose may be increased to 125 mg/kg-day, and to 6–8 g/day in adults (4). The optimal aspirin dose should ensure an adequate response but avoid toxicity. If symptoms of toxicity are present, they may subside after a few days despite continuation of the medication, but salicylate blood levels could be monitored if facilities are available (4, 5). After achieving the desired initial steady-state concentration for two weeks, the dosage can be decreased to 60–70 mg/kg-day for an additional

3–6 weeks (*2*, *4*, *5*). No controlled trials comparing aspirin and nonsteroidal anti-inflammatory agents have been conducted. However, in patients who are intolerant or allergic to aspirin, naproxen (10–20 mg/kg-day) has been used (*6*). One of the most common errors made by physicians is the early administration of anti-inflammatory therapy before the diagnosis has been finally established.

In a recent meta-analysis of salicylates and steroids, no differences were observed in the long-term outcomes of these treatments for decreasing the frequency of late rheumatic valvular disease (*7*). However, since one large study in the meta-analysis favoured the use of steroids, it remains unclear whether one treatment is superior to the other. Patients with pericarditis or heart failure respond favorably to corticosteroids; corticosteroids are also advisable in patients who do not respond to salicylates and who continue to worsen and develop heart failure despite anti-inflammatory therapy (*1*). Prednisone (1–2 mg/kg-day, to a maximum of 80 mg/day given once daily, or in divided doses) is usually the drug of choice. In life-threatening circumstances, therapy may be initiated with intravenous methyl prednisolone (*8*). After 2–3 weeks of therapy the dosage may be decreased by 20–25% each week (*2*, *5*). While reducing the steroid dosage, a period of overlap with aspirin is recommended to prevent rebound of disease activity (*1*, *9*).

Since there is no evidence that aspirin or corticosteroid therapy affects the course of carditis or reduces the incidence of subsequent heart disease, the duration of anti-inflammatory therapy is based upon the clinical response to therapy and normalization of acute phase reactants (*1*, *4*, *5*). Five per cent of patients continue to demonstrate evidence of rheumatic activity for six months or more, and may require a longer course of anti-inflammatory treatment (*4*). Infrequently, laboratory and clinical evidence of a rebound in disease activity may be noticed 2–3 weeks after stopping anti-inflammatory therapy (*4*). This usually resolves spontaneously and only severe symptoms require reinstitution of therapy (*4*).

Management of heart failure

Heart failure in RF generally responds to bed rest and steroids, but in patients with severe symptoms, diuretics, angiotensin converting enzyme inhibitors, and digoxin may be used (*4*, *5*, *10*). Initially, patients should follow a restricted sodium diet and diuretics should be administered. Angiotensin converting enzyme inhibitors and/or digoxin may be introduced if these measures are not effective, particularly in patients with advanced rheumatic valvular heart disease (*4*). No data exist on the use of angiotensin converting enzyme inhibitors to treat cardiac failure in children with RF. Their benefit has been extrapolated from trials in adults with congestive heart failure due to multiple etiologies (*10*).

Management of chorea

Chorea has traditionally been considered to be a self-limiting benign disease, requiring no therapy. However, there are recent reports that a protracted course can lead to disability and/or social isolation (*11*). The signs and symptoms of chorea generally do not respond well to anti-inflammatory agents. Neuroleptics, benzodiazepines and anti-epileptics are indicated, in combination with supportive measures such as rest in a quiet room. Haloperidol, diazepam, carbamazepine have all been reported to be effective in the treatment of chorea (*12–14*). There is no convincing evidence in the literature that steroids are beneficial for the therapy of the chorea associated with rheumatic fever.

References

1. Rheumatic fever and rheumatic heart disease. *Report of a WHO Expert Committee*. Geneva, World Health Organization, 1988 (WHO Technical Report Series, No. 764).

2. Silva NA, Pereira BA. Acute rheumatic fever: still a challenge. *Rheumatic Disease Clinic of North America*, 1997, **23**(3):545–568.

3. Tompkins DG, Boxerbaum B, Liebman J. Long-term prognosis of RF patients receiving regular intramuscular benzathine penicillin. *Circulation*, 1972, **45**:543–551.

4. Thatai D, Turi ZG. Current guidelines for the treatment of patients with rheumatic fever. *Drugs*, 1999, **57**(4):545–555.

5. Dajani AS. Rheumatic fever. In: Braunwald E, Zipes DP, Libby P, eds. *Heart Disease, 6th edition*, **2001**:2192–2198.

6. Uziel Y et al. The use of naproxen in the treatment of children with rheumatic fever. *Journal of Pediatrics*, 2000, **137**:269–271.

7. Daniel A et al. The treatment of rheumatic carditis: a review and meta-analyis. *Medicine*, 1995, **74**(1):1–12.

8. Herdy GV et al. Pulse therapy (high dose of venous methylprednisolone) in children with rheumatic carditis. Prospective study of 40 episodes. *Arquivos Brasileiros de Cardiologia*, 1993, **60**(6):377–381.

9. Feinstein AR, Spagnuolo M, Gill FA. Rebound phenomenon in acute rheumatic fever. I. Incidence and significance. *Yale Journal of Biological Medicine*, 1961, **33**:259–278.

10. Bonow RO, Carabello B, de Leon AC Jr. ACC/AHA guidelines for the management of patients with valvular heart disease. *Journal of the American College of Cardiology*, 1998, **32**:1486–1588.

11. **Swedo SE et al.** Sydenham's chorea: physical and psychological symptoms of St Vitus dance. *Pediatrics*, 1993, **91**:706–713.

12. **Mivakava M et al.** Effectiveness of haloperidol in the treatment of chorea minor. *Brain Development*, 1995, **27**:191–196.

13. **Zecharia HL et al.** Successful treatment of rheumatic chorea with carbamazepine. *Pediatric Neurology*, 2000, **23**(2):147–151.

14. **Ronchezel MV et al.** The use of haloperidol and valproate in children with Sydenham chorea. *Indian Pediatrics*, 1998, **35**(12):1215–1218.

9. Surgery for rheumatic heart disease

Surgery is usually performed for chronic rheumatic valve disease. It is rarely required during acute rheumatic fever (RF). In general terms, the necessity for surgical treatment is determined by the severity of the patient's symptoms and/or evidence that cardiac function is significantly impaired. It is particularly important to prevent irreversible damage to the left ventricle and irreversible pulmonary hypertension, since both considerably increase the risk of surgical treatment, impair long-term results and render surgery contra-indicated.

Indications for surgery in chronic valve disease

Echocardiography is essential for an assessment and follow-up of valvular disease. If echocardiography is not available, a diagnosis of valvular disease must rely on careful clinical examination supplemented by an electrocardiogram (ECG) and chest X-ray before the patient is referred to a cardiac surgical centre. Referrals for further assessment should be considered under the following circumstances (1, 2):

- Symptoms have progressed beyond New York Heart Association (NYHA) Class II. Note: with aortic stenosis (AS), *all* symptomatic patients should be referred.
- Patients who are asymptomatic, or mildly symptomatic, with progressive left ventricular enlargement on clinical or radiological examination (>0.5 cm/year).
- Cardiac failure due to the valve lesion itself, rather than to an episode of rheumatic carditis.
- Pulmonary hypertension, with physical signs and ECG evidence of changes in right ventricular hypertrophy, and chest X-ray evidence of pulmonary artery dilatation.
- Tricuspid regurgitation that complicates mitral valve disease.
- Development of atrial fibrillation.
- Thromboembolism.
- Endocarditis is suspected to contribute to cardiac decompensation.

Where facilities for echocardiography are available, regular assessments (at least once per year) should be undertaken. The following echocardiographic criteria should also be considered as indications for further assessment at a surgical centre, regardless of the patient's symptoms (1, 2):

Mitral stenosis (MS)

- Mitral valve area <1.5 cm^2 or valve area index <0.6 cm^2/m^2.
- The occurrence of dense, spontaneous echo contrast in the left atrium, because of the increased risk of thromboembolism.
- The presence of thrombus in the left atrial appendage or body of the left atrium.
- Pulmonary hypertension?

Mitral regurgitation (MR)

- Severe regurgitation on colour flow imaging.
- Left ventricular ejection fraction <50%.
- Left ventricular end-systolic dimension >55 mm.
- Pulmonary hypertension.

Aortic stenosis (AS)

- Valve area <0.8 cm^2 or valve area index <0.5 cm^2/m^2.
- Maximum jet velocity >4.0 m/sec.
- Left ventricular ejection fraction <50%.

Aortic regurgitation (AR)

- Severe regurgitation.
- Left ventricular ejection fraction <50%.
- Left ventricular end-systolic dimension >55 mm.

In patients with mitral and aortic valve disease, the threshold for referring symptomatic patients should be lower than each individual lesion would indicate.

The results of surgical treatment depend on: the severity of the disease process at the time of surgery; left ventricular function; nutritional status; and on long-term post-operative management, particularly anticoagulation management. Advanced NYHA functional class, impaired left ventricular function, atrial fibrillation, diabetes and other co-morbidities all have an adverse effect on hospital mortality rates and long-term survival rates (3). Operative mortality for elective, first-time single valve repair or replacement without any concomitant procedure is in the range of 2–5%. Further incremental increases in risk occur with emergency operations, re-operations, concomitant procedures such as coronary surgery, and operations for endocarditis (3, 4).

The indications for surgical treatment are as follows (1):

- In the presence of MS, patients with moderate or severe MS (mitral valve area 1.5 cm^2) and NYHA class II/IV symptoms.

- In the presence of MR, patients with NYHA functional class symptoms II/III/IV with:
  — normal left ventricular (LV) function (ejection fraction >60% and end-systolic dimension <45 mm);
  — mild dysfunction (ejection fraction 50–60% and end-systolic dimension 45–50 mm);
  — moderate dysfunction (ejection fraction 30–50% and end-systolic dimension 50–55 mm);
  — severe LV dysfunction and chordal preservation, or normal LV function and pulmonary hypertension.
- In the presence of AS, symptomatic patients with severe AS or in the presence of LV dysfunction, ventricular tachycardia, >15 mm LV hypertrophy, valve area <0.6 cm^2.
- In the presence of AR, with NYHA functional class symptoms II/III/IV with:
  — NYHA functional class III/IV and preserved LV function (ejection fraction >50%);
  — preserved LV function (ejection fraction >50%), but LV dilation or declining ejection fraction at rest or at functional studies;
  — mild dysfunction (ejection fraction 50–60% and end-systolic dimension 45–50 mm);
  — moderate dysfunction (ejection fraction 30–50% and end-systolic dimension 50–55 mm).

Contra-indications to surgery

There are few absolute contra-indications to valve surgery. Most are relative contra-indications and involve a risk/benefit calculation. Relative contra-indications include manifestations of end-stage valve disease, such as very poor LV function in association with a regurgitant lesion, severe fixed pulmonary hypertension or extensive extra-annular tissue destruction due to uncontrolled endocarditis. Poor LV function in association with isolated severe AS is rarely a contra-indication, as considerable improvement can be expected following relief of the obstruction. Judgment is often more difficult when severe AS coexists with extensive coronary disease and the cause of the LV dysfunction is uncertain.

The age of the patient and the presence of co-morbidities also affect risk/benefit calculations. Young patients often have a remarkable capacity for recovery, even from end-stage valve disease. Conversely, adverse risk factors have a much more pronounced effect in older patients. Co-morbidities that require consideration include:

— renal failure (particularly if local facilities for haemofiltration or haemodialysis are scarce);
— advanced pulmonary disease;
— severe haemolytic anaemia which can not be controlled medically;
— severe generalized arteriopathy;
— malignant diseases;
— extreme overweight (leading to pulmonary complications);
— serious infections until they can be eradicated.

Good nutritional status improves post-operative chances of survival, while severe cachexia due to cardiac or other causes greatly reduces the chances of survival.

Treatment options

Balloon valvotomy (commissurotomy)

This technique is reserved almost entirely for stenosis of the mitral valve. Overall, the incidence of re-stenosis is reported to be about 40% after seven years (5), although this may vary according to the population studied (6). In some cases, it is feasible to repeat the procedure if re-stenosis is confined to commissural fusion only. In low resource settings, the cost of the procedure means it is not an optimal choice.

Surgical treatment

Surgical procedures performed include closed mitral commissuro-tomy, valve repair and valve replacement. Valve repair techniques and valve replacement require open-heart surgery using cardiopul-monary bypass. Valve repair to prevent progression of rheumatic valvular disease is not indicated (7). Also, although a bioprosthetic valve may be appealing for young women who wish to become pregnant, it may deteriorate more rapidly during pregnancy, particularly with multiple pregnancies (8, 9). In many developing countries, the use of biological and bioprosthetic valves has almost been abandoned, and mechanical valves represent the best compromise for young and middle-aged patients with rheumatic valve disease, despite the need for long-term anticoagulation treatment (10). In fact, the risk of thromboembolism in young active patients in sinus rhythm with good LV function is much lower than that of the typical older middle-aged and elderly valve patients with associated risk factors such as diabetes, hypertension and arterial disease (11, 12). It is important that the least thrombogenic prostheses be implanted, since it can be difficult to manage long-term anticoagulation therapy in low-resource settings. In general, mechanical valves with a bileaflet design seem more prone to valve thrombosis if anticoagulation is not used, or if the treatment is suboptimal, compared to valves with a modern tilting disc design (*11–13*).

Long-term complications

Long-term complications of valve replacement include (*13*):

— structural valve deterioration (this is only a concern for biological and bioprosthetic valves and the deterioration is time-dependent);
— valve thrombosis (0.01–0.5% per year);
— thromboembolism (2–5% per year);
— prosthetic endocarditis (0.2–1.2% per year);
— major bleeding (conventionally attributed to anticoagulation), 1–4% per year;
— paravalvular leak (0.1–1.5% per year).

Many of these complications, particularly valve thrombosis, thromboembolism, endocarditis and bleeding, are related more to patient and management factors than to the prosthesis itself. The need to replace prosthetic valves tends to be higher in developing countries because of difficulties in post-operative management, and because prosthetic valves need to be replaced in growing children.

Long-term postoperative management

All patients who have undergone intervention treatment for rheumatic valve disease will require regular long-term follow-up (*1*). Ideally, this should be done in a centre equipped with echocardiography. Patients who have had conservative valve procedures, such as valvotomy or valve repair, require close observation to detect re-stenosis or a recurrence of valve regurgitation, and to ensure secondary prophylaxis. It is also important to monitor LV function and prosthetic function.

If echocardiography is not available, patients should be referred back to the surgical centre if they develop any of the following:

— recurrent symptoms
— evidence of cardiac failure
— muffled prosthetic heart sounds
— a new regurgitant murmur
— any thromboembolic episode
— symptoms and signs suggestive of endocarditis.

Any of the above conditions may indicate a complication related to the prosthesis, and all require further investigation (*14*). If only one valve has been repaired or replaced, progression of valve disease at another site may also be a cause of patient deterioration.

In patients with mechanical valves, anticoagulation control is the most important, independent determinant of long-term survival (*14, 15*), and is perhaps the most important aspect of post-operative management. Good anticoagulation management has three principal components (*16*):

1. Standardized anticoagulation measurement, using the International Normalised Ratio (INR).
2. Prosthesis-specific and patient-specific anticoagulation intensity. In general terms, a patient with a low-thrombogenicity prosthesis in the aortic position, who is in sinus rhythm and has good LV function can be managed with an INR in the range 2.5–3.0, whereas a patient with a low-thrombogenicity prosthesis in the mitral position, or who is in atrial fibrillation, or has impaired LV function, will need a higher INR (in the range 3.0–3.5). Patients with more-thrombogenic prostheses may require an INR in the range 3.5–4.0. However, it must emphasized that ideal INR ranges have yet to be determined for all currently available prosthetic valves.
3. Regular monitoring of the INR and maintaining it within the therapeutic range. In developing countries, small portable devices for monitoring INR may have a role in remote communities, where an experienced health worker can monitor the INR of many patients within a particular community (*17*).

Long-term management also involves regular penicillin prophylaxis in high-risk patients, to prevent further episodes of RF (*18*). Endocarditis prophylaxis is also necessary to cover any dental or surgical procedure. It is essential that patients and their relatives are fully informed about the importance of endocarditis prophylaxis, as many studies report a mortality rate from prosthetic endocarditis of >50% (*19*). Refer to Chapter 11, *Infective endocarditis*, for a discussion of endocarditis prophylaxis.

The role of surgery in active rheumatic carditis

Traditional belief has discouraged the surgical option in acute RF, given the profound inflammatory state. An earlier study series (*20*) showed that repair or replacement surgery was possible in mitral valve disease (stenotic or regurgitant), albeit with a high rate of in-hospital mortality. Of 304 instances of mitral valve replacement or repair in patients with mitral valve disease of rheumatic etiology, the total hospital mortality rate was 3.2%, but was as high as 19.2% if valve replacement was performed after a failed attempt at repair. Of the 26 reoperations, 24 needed the second procedure owing to mitral valve dysfunction, and 8 of 24 patients had active rheumatic carditis. The actuarial total survival at 30 months was 72% for valve replacement and 94% for valve repair. The authors stressed the need for better preoperative identification of valvular lesions, using techniques such as echocardiography (*21*) to prevent unsuccessful attempts at valvular repair. Details of the rheumatic carditis patients were not available from this study, and other studies reporting less-favorable outcomes are only anecdotal.

However, after the series published by Essop and co-workers (*22*), there was a change in how the surgical option was viewed. In the series, 32 patients with medically refractory acute carditis and congestive heart failure (CHF) underwent mitral or mitral and aortic valve replacement. There was no operative mortality and there was a significant decrease in the heart size and resolution of heart failure. Ventricular contractile function was preserved, and there was no mortality or decline in ventricular function during the follow-up period. This study established that surgery was a preferred option over the long-term use of high-dose corticosteroids for severe refractory acute carditis, and also disproved that a "myocardial factor" played a role in the pathogenesis of acute RF. Since contractility parameters were preserved and returned to the normal range after the valvular lesion was corrected (even in the most severe cases), this discounted any notion of a significant myocardial component to the clinical picture. This was also borne out by echocardiographic studies that evaluated ventricular mechanics during acute RF, and which found that cardiac function remained stable throughout the course of the disease, despite the presence of CHF (*23*). Endomyocardial biopsies performed during the acute phase of the disease failed to demonstrate evidence of myocardial damage, and inflammatory activity was confined to the interstitial compartment only (*24*). The resolution of CHF after valvular surgery also suggested that the pathophysiological derangement seen in acute RF was caused by valvular regurgitation secondary to valvulitis.

In a subsequent study, 254 patients (aged 6–52 years) with pure rheumatic regurgitant lesion and CHF (96% in NYHA class III or IV) were enrolled in a study to examine the efficacy of repairing the mitral valve surgically (*25*). Of the 254 patients, 76 showed acute rheumatic activity. The patients were followed for 60 ± 35 months after surgery. The acute mortality rate for the patients was 2.6% and the five-year mortality rate was 15%. There was a high incidence of valve failure, which necessitated reoperation (27%). The presence of acute carditis correlated with reoperations, and patients undergoing "early" reoperations were more likely to have rheumatic activity (47%)

compared to those with "late" reoperations. The mean event free survival at five years was 73%. Thus, surgical valve repair during active carditis was associated with an acceptable survival rate, but reoperations were frequent.

From the available studies, the following observations can be made(20–25):

- Surgery can be safely performed during active carditis and, in refractory cases of active carditis, may be preferable to the long-term use of corticosteroids.
- Myocardial inflammation plays no significant role in the clinical pathology of active carditis.
- Valve repair during active carditis may not constitute the best surgical option if there is macroscopic evidence of valvular inflammation, because valve repair is associated with significant reoperation rates.

References

1. Bonow RO et al. ACC/AHA guidelines for the management of patients with valvular heart disease. *Journal of the American College of Cardiology*, 1998, 32:1486–1588.

2. Jamieson WRE et al. Risk stratification for cardiac valve replacement. National Cardiac Surgery Database. *Annals of Thoracic Surgery*, 1999, 67:943–951.

3. Lindblom D et al. Long-term relative survival rates after heart valve replacement. *Journal of the American College of Cardiology*, 1990, 15:566–578.

4. Gometza B et al. Surgery for rheumatic mitral regurgitation below twenty years of age. An analysis of failures. *Journal of Heart Valve Disease*, 1996, 5:294–301.

5. Mohamed Ben F et al. Percutaneous balloon versus surgical closed and open mitral commissurotomy: seven year follow-up results of a randomized trail. *Circulation*, 1998, 971:245–250.

6. Yau TM et al. Mitral valve repair and replacement for rheumatic disease. *Journal of Thoracic and Cardiovascular Surgery*, 2000, 119:53–61.

7. Sbarouni E, Oakley CM. Outcome of pregnancy in women with valve prostheses. *British Heart Journal*, 1994, 71:196–201.

8. North RA et al. Long-term survival and valve-related complications in young women with cardiac valve replacement. *Circulation*, 1999, 99:2669–2676.

9. Hammermeister K et al. Outcomes 15 years after valve replacement with a mechanical versus a bioprosthetic valve: final report of the Veteran Affairs randomised trial. *Journal of the American College of Cardiology*, 2000, 36:1152–1153.

10. **Butchart EG et al.** The role of risk factors and trigger factors in cerebrovascular events after mitral valve replacement. *Journal of Cardiac Surgery*, 1994, **9**(Suppl.):228–236.

11. **Butchart EG.** Prosthetic heart valves. In: *Cardiovascular thrombosis*, 2nd ed. Verstraete M, Fuster V, Topol EJ, eds. Philadelphia, Lippincott-Raven, **1998**:399–418.

12. **Butchart EG et al.** Arterial risk factors and cerebrovascular events following aortic valve replacement. *Journal of Heart Valve Disease*, 1995, 4:1–8.

13. **Grunkemeier GL et al.** Long-term performance of prosthetic heart valves. *Current Problems in Cardiology*, 2000, **25**:73–156.

14. **Butchart EG et al.** Better anticoagulation control improves survival after valve replacement. *Journal of Thoracic and Cardiovascular Surgery*. (In press).

15. **Gohlke-Bärwolf C et al.** Guidelines for prevention of thromboembolic events in valvular heart disease. Study Group of the Working Group on Valvular Heart Disease of the European Society of Cardiology. *European Heart Journal*, 1995, **16**:1320–1330.

16. **Taborski U, Müller-Berghaus G.** State-of-the-art patient self-management for control of oral anticoagulation. *Seminars in Thrombosis and Hemostatics*, 1999, **25**:43–47.

17. **Dajani AS et al.** Prevention of bacterial endocarditis: recommendations of the American Heart Association. *Circulation*, 1997, **96**:358–366.

18. **Bayer AS et al.** Diagnosis and management of infective endocarditis and its complications. *Circulation*, 1998, **98**:2936–2948.

19. **Moon MR et al.** Surgical treatment of endocarditis. *Progress in Cardiovascular Disease*, 1997, **40**:239–264.

20. **Duran CM, Gometza B, de Vol EB.** Valve repair in rheumatic mitral disease. *Circulation*, 1991, **84**(5 Suppl.):III125–132.

21. **Vasan RS et al.** Echocardiographic evaluation of patients with acute rheumatic fever and rheumatic carditis. *Circulation*, 1996, **94**(1):73–82.

22. **Essop MR, Wisenbaugh T, Sareli P.** Evidence against a myocardial factor as the cause of left ventricular dilation in active rheumatic carditis. *Journal of the American College of Cardiology*, 1993, **22**(3):826–829.

23. **Gentles TL et al.** Left ventricular mechanics during and after acute rheumatic fever: contractile dysfunction is closely related to valve regurgitation. *Journal of the American College of Cardiology*, 2001, **37**(1):201–207.

24. **Narula J et al.** Does endomyocardial biopsy aid in the diagnosis of active rheumatic carditis. *Circulation*, 1993, **88**(5 Pt. 1):2198–2205.

25. **Skoularigis J et al.** Evaluation of the long-term results of mitral valve repair in 254 young patients with rheumatic mitral regurgitation. *Circulation*, 1994, **90**(5 Pt 2):II167–174.

10. **Primary prevention of rheumatic fever**

The primary prevention of rheumatic fever (RF) is defined as the adequate antibiotic therapy of group A streptococcal upper respiratory tract (URT) infections to prevent an initial attack of acute RF (*1–9*). Primary prevention is administered only when there is group A streptococcal URT infection. The therapy is therefore intermittent, in contrast to the therapy used for the secondary prevention of RF, where antibiotics are administered continuously (see table 12.7).

Epidemiology of group A streptococcal upper respiratory tract infection

Group A streptococcal infection is endemic throughout the world, but sporadic epidemics are common, particularly among schoolchildren, in residential facilities for the elderly, and in other unique populations such as military personnel. Although group A streptococcal colonization and infection of the URT is common and can occur in people of any age, streptococcal pharyngitis/tonsillitis primarily affects children between the ages of 5–15 years. It is thought that natural immunity can be conferred by the surface M-protein of specific group A streptococci (M-types), but since more than 130 different M-proteins have been described, it is common for individuals throughout their lifetime to have multiple infections by different M-type streptococci.

Group A streptococcal URT infections can lead to RF and acute post-streptococcal glomerulonephritis. In contrast, although some have proposed otherwise, group A streptococcal skin infections do not appear to predispose to acute RF, but can lead to post-streptococcal glomerulonephritis.

Diagnosis of group A streptococcal pharyngitis

To treat patients effectively and prevent suppurative and non-suppurative sequelae, it is important that group A streptococcal pharyngitis be diagnosed promptly and accurately. An accurate and prompt diagnosis will not only help to control the spread of infection, it will also minimize the inappropriate use of antibiotics. The inappropriate use of antibiotics is a consideration because most cases of pharyngitis are caused by viruses, and of the many bacterial pathogens that cause pharyngitis (Table 10.1), antibiotic therapy is only recommended for group A streptococcal infection (with rare exceptions). Indeed, cases of group A streptococcal pharingytis represent only 20% of all pharyngitis cases (*9*).

It is often difficult to diagnose streptococcal URT infection, even for experienced clinicians, despite the fact that the clinical symptoms

Table 10.1
The most common bacterial causes of pharyngitis[a]

Organism	Illness
Streptococcus pyogenes (Group A)	Pharyngitis and tonsillitis
Streptococcus pyogenes (Group C or G)	Pharyngitis and tonsillitis
Neisseria gonorrheae	Pharyngitis
Corynebacterium diphtheria	Diphtheria
Arcanobacterium hemolyticum	Pharyngitis

[a] Modified from (*10*).

associated with such an infection occur frequently. The complex of symptoms include a sudden onset of high fever, very sore throat with dysphagia, a scarlatiniform rash and abdominal pain. Numerous attempts have been made to devise algorithms to make the clinical diagnosis easier (especially in areas where a microbiology laboratory is not available), but in general these algorithms lack accuracy and are not universally helpful. Part of the difficulty in devising an algorithm derives from the fact most common clinical findings associated with group A streptococcal URT infection can differ by age of the patient. Examples of the most frequently observed clinical findings, signs and symptoms are shown for different age groups in Table 10.2.

No single element of history taking or physical examination is accurate enough to exclude or diagnose streptococcal throat infection. Patient factors such as age younger than 15 years, history of fever, tonsillar swelling or exudate, tender anterior cervical lymphadenopathy and absence of cough should all be taken into consideration in arriving at a diagnosis. If four or five of the factors are present, the likelihood ratio of streptococcal infection is 4.9 (approximately 50% of cases); if 3 factors are present the ratio decreases to 2.5 (approximately 25%); and if only 2 are present, to 0.9 (approximately 10%) (*12*).

Laboratory diagnosis

Since the clinical diagnosis of acute streptococcal pharyngitis is often imprecise, laboratory confirmation is needed, although in many parts of the world clinical laboratory facilities are not available (*7, 8, 11, 12*). A major function of a clinical laboratory in the diagnosis and management of group A streptococcal URT infections are to culture throat samples and, when available, to perform rapid antigen detection tests. The throat culture is optimal for confirming whether there are group A streptococci in the URT of patients with acute pharyngitis. If carried out properly, the sensitivity and specificity of this assay

Table 10.2
Clinical signs and symptoms of group A streptococcal upper respiratory tract infection, by patient age group[a]

Clinical signs and/or symptoms	Infants	School-age children	Adolescents and adults
Anterior cervical lymphadenitis (tender nodes)	++++[b]	++++	++++
Close contact with an infected person	++++	++++	++++
Scarlatiniform rash	Unusual	++++	++++
Excoriated nares	++++	Unusual	Unusual
Tonsillar or pharyngeal exudate	Uncommon in infants younger than three years of age	++++	++++
Positive throat culture	++++	++++	++++
Fever	++ (Not specific)	++ (Not specific)	++ (Not specific)
Acute onset of symptoms	+ (Unusual)	++ (Not specific)	++ (Not specific)
Abdominal pain	++	++	+ (Unusual)
Coryza	++	Unusual	Unusual
Erythema of the pharynx	Not specific	Not specific	Not specific
Hoarseness	Unusual	Unusual	Unusual
Cough	Unusual	Unusual	Unusual

[a] Modified from (11).
[b] The symptoms are classified semiquantitatively as being: less typical (+); more typical and frequent/moderately suggestive (++); and almost always present in patients with streptococcal pharyngitis/very suggestive (++++).

are excellent (see Chapter 5, *The role of the microbiology laboratory in the diagnosis of streptococcal infections and rheumatic fever*). Rapid antigen detection tests are available in some parts of the world, and almost exclusively use antibodies directed against the group A carbohydrate of the streptococcal cell wall. The specificity of the immunoassays most often exceeds their sensitivity. In general, they are more expensive than blood agar plates, and like culture plates they need refrigeration, which can be a problem in some parts of the world, especially those with tropical climates.

Group A streptococcal antibodies to extracellular antigens such as streptolysin-O (antistreptolysin-O) or deoxyribonuclease B (anti-DNase B) have little or no use in diagnosing acute group A streptococcal pharyngitis or tonsillitis, since they can be accurately interpreted only in retrospect. This should not detract from their importance in assisting with the diagnosis of acute RF, however, which requires evidence of a preceding group A streptococcal infection (see the Jones Criteria in Chapter 3, *Diagnosis of rheumatic fever*). If laboratory facilities are not available, a diagnosis of streptococcal pharyngitis has to be made on the basis of clinical findings (*7, 8, 11–13*).

Antibiotic therapy of group A streptococcal pharyngitis

Effective antibiotic therapy *eradicates* group A streptococci from the URT and can prevent RF if therapy is started within nine days after the onset of symptoms (*1, 3, 9, 13*). Table 10.3 shows the most commonly used antibiotics to treat group A streptococcal URT infections. To date, no clinical isolate of group A beta-hemolytic streptococcus (*Streptococcus pyogenes*) has been shown to be resistant to penicillin. For this reason, and because penicillin is inexpensive and available in most countries, it remains the drug of choice for treating group A streptococcal URT infections (*14–24*). To eradicate a group A streptococcal infection, oral penicillin (penicillin V or penicillin G) should be given for a full 10 days (*25–29*). A single intramuscular injection of benzathine benzylpenicillin can be used to treat the infection if it is anticipated that the patient will not adhere to a treatment regimen of oral antibiotics. First-generation cephalosporins have also been used successfully. In contrast, tetracyclines and sulfa drugs are contraindicated for the primary prevention of RF because many group A streptococci are resistant.

For patients with allergies to penicillin, the macrolide erythromycin has been the recommended antibiotic of choice for many years. However, in the 1960s and 1970s, the prevalence of macrolide-resistant group A streptococci began to increase in areas where macrolides were widely used, to the point that it became a clinically significant problem (e.g. in several countries in Europe) (*30–32*). In many countries, resistance to macrolide antibiotics has reached more than 15%. This must be taken into account when considering a macrolide for therapy of group A streptococcal URT infection. In some cases, the increase in resistance has been related to the introduction of new macrolide drugs that frequently are recommended only for abbreviated therapy. Shortened courses of antibiotic therapy remain controversial since there is a paucity of carefully conducted studies to confirm that this form of therapy is fully effective in eradicating group A streptococci from the URT (*24, 32, 33*).

Most authorities do not believe that routine culturing of the patient's throat after completing antibiotic therapy is indicated, except in unique epidemiological situations such as a patient known to have RF or rheumatic heart disease (*9*).

Table 10.3
Primary prevention of rheumatic fever: recommended treatment for streptococcal pharyngitis[a,b]

Antibiotic	Administration	Dose	Comments
Benzathine benzylpenicillin	Single intramuscular injection	1 200 000 units intramuscularly; 600 000 units for children weighing <27 kg.	Preferable to oral penicillin because of patient adherence problems.
Phenoxymethyl penicillin (Penicillin V)	Orally 2–4 times/day for 10 full days	Children: 250 mg bid or tid. Adolescents or adults: 250 mg tid or qid, or 500 mg bid.	Penicillin resistance by group A streptococci has never been reported.
Amoxicillin	Orally 2–3 times/day for 10 full days	25–50 mg/kg/day in three doses. Total adult dose is 750–1500 mg/day.	Acceptable alternative to oral penicillin because of the taste.
First-generation cephalosporins[c]	Orally 2–3 times/day for 10 full days	Varies with agent.	Acceptable alternative for oral penicillin.[d]
Erythromycin ethylsuccinate	Orally 4 times/day for 10 full days	Varies with formulation. Available as the stearate, ethylsuccinate, estolate or base.	Alternative drug for patients allergic to penicillin. Should not be used in areas where group A streptococci have high rates of macrolide resistance.

[a] Modified in part from (24).
[b] In some countries, macrolides have been approved for an abbreviated course of therapy (shorter than 10 days), but the efficacy of this treatment is controversial and it cannot be recommended at presen:. Also, trimethoprim, sulfonamides and tetracyclines are not effective antibiotics for eradicating Group A streptococci and are not indicated for the primary prevention of RF.
[c] These agents should not be used in patients who have had immediate-type hypersensitivity to beta-lactam antibiotics.
[d] This has been used in some patients who have either a poorly documented history of penicillin allergy, but should not be used for patients with immediate hypersensitivity reactions to penicillin (e.g. anaphylaxis or hives). About 5% of those who have even a mild allergic reaction to penicillin may also have a reaction to cephalosporins.

Special situations

If pharyngitis recurs after antibiotic therapy has been completed it will be necessary to perform a throat culture to confirm that group A streptococci are responsible. M-typing of strains when possible may be necessary to establish whether the recurrence was because of treatment failure or because of a new infection. The same antibiotic used to treat the infection initially should be administered, especially if a new infection is suspected. If oral penicillin had been used initially, then a single intramuscular injection is recommended. If it is suspected that the streptococci are penicillinase producers it is advisable to administer clindamycin or amoxycillin/clavulanate (*9, 26, 34–36*).

Antibiotics should not be administered to group A streptococcal carriers, because they are unlikely to spread the microorganism to contacts and they are at a low risk, if any, of developing RF (*9, 37*).

Other primary prevention approaches

Although a cost-effective vaccine for group A streptococci would be the ideal solution, scientific problems have prevented the development of such a vaccine (see Chapter 13, *Prospects for a streptococcal vaccine*). There have been no controlled studies showing that tonsillectomy is effective in reducing the incidence of RF, and it is not recommended for the primary prevention of RF (*24, 28, 38–40*).

References

1. **Denny F et al.** Prevention of rheumatic fever. Treatment of the preceding streptococcal infection. *Journal of the American Medical Association*, 1950, 143:151–153.

2. **Wannamaker LW et al.** Prophylaxis of acute rheumatic fever by treatment of the preceding streptococcal infection with various amount of depot penicillin. *American Journal of Medicine*, 1951, 10:673–695.

3. **Gordis L.** The virtual disappearance of rheumatic fever in the United States: lessons in the rise and fall of disease. *Circulation*, 1985, 72(6):1155.

4. **Markowwitz M, Kaplan EL.** Reappearance of rheumatic fever. *Advances in Pediatrics*, 1989, 36:39–65.

5. **Kaplan EL, Hill HR.** Return of rheumatic fever: consequences, implications, and needs. *Journal of Pediatrics*, 1987, 111(2):244–246.

6. **Dodu SRA, Bothig S.** Rheumatic fever and rheumatic heart disease in developing countries. *World Health Forum*, 1989, 10(2):203–212.

7. *Joint WHO/ISFC meeting on RF/RHD control with emphasis on primary prevention, Geneva, 7–9 September 1994.* Geneva, World Health Organization, 1994 (WHO Document WHO/CVD 94.1).

8. *The WHO Global Programme for the prevention of RF/RHD. Report of a consultation to review progress and develop future activities.* Geneva, World Health Organization, 2000 (WHO document WHO/CVD/00.1).

9. **Bisno AL et al.** Practice guidelines for the diagnosis and management of group A streptococcal pharyngitis. *Clinical Infectious Diseases*, 2002, **35**(2):113–125.

10. **Bisno AL.** Acute pharyngitis: etiology and diagnosis. *Pediatrics*, 1996, **97**(6 Pt 2):949–954.

11. **Wannamaker LW.** Perplexity and precision in the diagnosis of streptococcal pharyngitis. *American Journal of Diseases of Children*, 1972, **124**(3):352–358.

12. **Ebell MH et al.** The rational clinical examination. Does this patient have strep throat? *Journal of the American Medical Association*, 2000, **284**(22):2912–2918.

13. **Shet A, Kaplan EL.** Clinical use and interpretation of group A streptococcal antibody tests: a practical approach for the pediatrician or primary care physician. *Pediatric Infectious Disease Journal*, 2002, **21**(5):420–430.

14. **Stollerman GH.** Penicillin for streptococcal pharyngitis: has anything changed? *Hospital Practice*, 1995, **30**(3):80–83.

15. **Krause RM.** Prevention of streptococcal sequelae by penicillin prophylaxis: a reassessment. *Journal of Infectious Diseases*, 1975, **131**(5):592–601.

16. **Dajani AS.** Rheumatic fever prevention revisited. *Pediatric Infectious Disease Journal,* 1989, **8**(5):266–267.

17. **Markowitz M.** Benzathine penicillin G after thirty years. *Clinical therapeutics*, 1980, **3**(1):49–61.

18. **Pichichero ME.** Eradication of group A streptococci. *Pediatrics*, 2000, **106**(2 Pt 1):380–382.

19. **El Kholy A.** A controlled study of penicillin therapy of group A streptococcal acquisitions in Egyptian families. *Journal of Infectious Diseases*, 1980, **141**(6):759–771.

20. **Bass JW.** A review of the rationale and advantages of various mixtures of benzathine penicillin G. *Pediatrics*, 1996, **97**(6 Pt 2):960–963.

21. **Bass JW et al.** Streptococcal pharyngitis in children. A comparison of four treatment schedules with intramuscular penicillin G benzathine. *Journal of the American Medical Association*, 1976, **235**(11):1112–1126.

22. **Feldman S et al.** Efficacy of benzathine penicillin G in group A streptococcal pharyngitis: reevaluation. *Journal of Pediatrics*, 1987, **110**(5):783–787.

23. **Massel BF.** Prevention of rheumatic fever. *Journal of the American Medical Association*, 1972, **221**(4):410–411.

24. *WHO model prescribing information. Drugs used in the treatment of streptococcal pharyngitis and prevention of rheumatic fever.* Geneva, World Health Organization, 1999 (WHO/EDM/PAR/99.1).

25. **Pichichero ME et al.** Variables influencing penicillin treatment outcome in streptococcal tonsillopharyngitis. *Archives of Pediatrics and Adolescent Medicine*, 1999, **153**(6):565–570.

26. **Smith TD et al.** Efficacy of beta-lactamase-resistant penicillin and influence of penicillin tolerance in eradicating streptococci from the pharynx after failure of penicillin therapy for group A streptococcal pharyngitis. *Journal of Pediatrics*, 1987, **110**(5):777–782.

27. **Kaplan EL, Johnson J.** Eradication of group A streptococci from the upper respiratory tract by amoxicillin with clavulanate after oral penicillin V treatment failure. *Journal of Pediatrics*, 1988, **113**(2):400–403.

28. **Matanoski GM et al.** Epidemiology of streptococcal infections in rheumatic and non-rheumatic families. IV. The effect of tonsillectomy on streptococcal infections. *American Journal of Epidemiology*, 1968, **87**(1):226–236.

29. **Venuta A et al.** Azithromycin compared with clarithromycin for the treatment of streptococcal pharyngitis in children. *Journal of International Medical Research*, 1998, **26**(3):152–158.

30. **Gerber MA et al.** Potemtial mechanisms for failure to eradicate group A streptococci from the pharynx. *Pediatrics*, 1999, **104**(4):911–917.

31. **Kaplan EL, Johnson DR.** Unexplained reduced microbiological efficacy of intramuscular benzathine penicillin G and oral penicillin V in eradication of group A streptococci from children with acute pharyngitis. *Pediatrics*, 2001, **108**(5):1180–1186.

32. **Shulman ST.** Evaluation of penicillins, cephalosporins and macrolides for therapy of streptococcal pharyngitis. *Pediatrics*, 1996, **97**:955–959.

33. **Zwart S et al.** Penicillin for acute sore throat: randomized double blind trial of seven days versus three days treatment or placebo in adults. *British Medical Journal*, 2000, **320**:150–154.

34. **Chaudhary S et al.** Penicillin V and rifampin for the treatment of group A streptococcal pharyngitis: a randomized trial of 10 days penicillin vs 10 days penicillin with rifampin during the final 4 days of therapy. *Journal of Pediatrics*, 1985, **106**(3):481–486.

35. **Orrling A et al.** Clindamycin in persisting streptococcal pharyngotonsillitis after penicillin treatment. *Scandinavian Journal of Infectious Diseases*, 1994, **26**(5):535–541.

36. **Tanz RR et al.** Penicillin plus rifampin eradicates pharyngeal carriage of group A streptococci. *Journal of Pediatrics*, 1985, **106**(6):876–880.

37. **Cremer EJ et al.** Azithromycin versus cefaclor in the treatment of pediatric patients with acute group A beta-hemolytic streptococcal tonsillopharyngitis. *European Journal of Clinical Microbiology and Infectious Diseases*, 1998, **17**(4):235–239.

38. **Matanoski GM.** The role of the tonsils in streptococcal infections: a comparison of tonsillectomized children and sibling controls. *American Journal of Epidemiology*, 1972, **95**(3):278–291.

39. **Paradise JL et al.** Efficacy of tonsillectomy for recurrent throat infection in severely affected children. Results of parallel randomized and

nonrandomized clinical trials. *New England Journal of Medicine*, 1984, **310**(11):674–683.

40. **Walsh H, Dowd B.** Tonsillectomy and rheumatic fever. *Medical Journal of Australia*, 1967, **2**(25):1121–1123.

11. Secondary prevention of rheumatic fever

Definition of secondary prevention

Secondary prevention of rheumatic fever (RF) is defined as the continuous administration of specific antibiotics to patients with a previous attack of RF, or a well-documented rheumatic heart disease (RHD). The purpose is to prevent colonization or infection of the upper respiratory tract (URT) with group A beta-hemolytic streptococci and the development of recurrent attacks of RF. Secondary prophylaxis is mandatory for all patients who have had an attack of RF, whether or not they have residual rheumatic valvular heart disease.

Antibiotics used for secondary prophylaxis: general principles

Intramuscular injection of benzathine benzylpenicillin every three weeks (every four weeks in low-risk areas or low risk patients) is the most effective strategy for preventing recurrent attacks of RF (*1*). Oral penicillin may also be used as an alternative in secondary prophylaxis, but the greatest concern with oral administration is noncompliance, since patients often find it difficult to adhere to a daily regimen of antibiotics for many years (*2*). Even for patients who strictly adhere to the regimen, serum penicillin levels are less predictable with this method, and RF recurs more frequently in patients on an oral regimen than in comparable patients receiving intramuscular benzathine benzylpenicillin (*3*). Situations in which an oral regimen may be used include patients who are at a relatively low risk for a recurrence of RF, and those who refuse to accept the regular injection schedule.

Penicillin remains the antibiotic of choice (*4*). For those patients who are known to be, or are suspected of being, allergic to penicillin, oral sulfadiazine or oral sulfasoxazole represent optimal second choices (*5*). In the rare instance where patients are allergic both to penicillin and the sulfa drugs, or if these drugs are not available, oral erythromycin may be used (*5*). Note that while the sulfa drugs should not be used for primary prophylaxis, they are acceptable for secondary prophylaxis. A complete list of antibiotics and appropriate dosage schedules for the secondary prophylaxis of recurrent RF is provided in Table 11.1.

Benzathine benzylpenicillin

Benzathine benzylpenicillin is a repository form of penicillin G designed to provide a sustained bactericidal serum concentration. Early studies indicated that serum levels of penicillin remained above the

Table 11.1
Antibiotics used in secondary prophylaxis of RF

Antibiotic	Mode of administration	Dose
Benzathine benzylpenicillin	Single intramuscular injection every 3–4 weeks.	For adults and children ≥30 kg in weight: 1 200 000 units. For children <30 kg in weight: 600 000 units.
Penicillin V.	Oral.	250 mg twice daily.
Sulfonamide (e.g. sulfadiazine, sulfadoxine, sulfisoxazole).	Oral.	For adults and children ≥30 kg in weight: 1 gram daily. For children <30 kg in weight: 500 mg daily.
Erythromycin.	Oral.	250 mg twice daily.

Modified in part from (5)

minimum inhibitory concentration for group A streptococci for 3–4 weeks (6). Vials of the antibiotic usually contain 1.2 million units, equivalent to 720 mg of benzyl penicillin G. The reconstituted or lyophilized penicillin should be stored at temperatures not exceeding 30 °C and be protected from moisture. Although the activity of benzathine benzylpenicillin remains stable in the vial for several years if appropriately stored, the activity may be affected by the presence of preservatives (4). The physical properties of the solution, if not optimal, may also affect its degree of solubility and hence its absorption from the injection site, which can affect its bioavailability (7). Since preparations of benzathine benzylpenicillin are available from pharmaceutical manufacturers around the world, quality control procedures are necessary to ensure that the preparations have optimal absorption characteristics and that effective serum levels of penicillin will be maintained between injections.

After deep intramuscular injection, peak serum concentrations are usually reached within 12–24 hours and effective concentrations are usually detectable for approximately three weeks in most patients and for four weeks in a smaller proportion (8). The usual dose for secondary RF prophylaxis is 1.2 million units given intramuscularly, most often administered in the upper outer quadrant of the buttock, or in the anterior lateral thigh.

Oral penicillin

Although published data indicate that intramuscular benzathine benzylpenicillin is superior to oral penicillin for preventing acquisition of group A beta-hemolytic streptococci in the URT, and for preventing subsequent recurrences of acute RF, oral regimens can be used.

Originally, oral regimens utilized penicillin G, but this is more susceptible to gastric hydrolysis than penicillin V. Since penicillin V is now as inexpensive as penicillin G, and since penicillin V is available in most countries, it is the preferred form of oral penicillin. The usual dose is 250 mg taken twice daily (Table 11.1).

Oral sulfadiazine or sulfasoxazole

For a patient allergic to penicillin, oral sulfadiazine or sulfasoxazole are acceptable substitutes, unless the patient is also sensitive to sulfa drugs (5). These drugs are also contraindicated in pregnancy. Although sulfa drugs are effective in preventing colonization of the URT with group A beta-hemolytic streptococci, they *cannot* be used for the primary prevention of established streptococcal infections. The dose is either one gram daily or 500 mg daily, depending on the weight of the patient (Table 11.1).

Duration of secondary prophylaxis

It is difficult to formulate "blanket" guidelines for the duration of secondary prophylaxis. The duration of prophylaxis for a patient with a questionable history of RF and no evidence of valvular heart disease, for example, may be different than that for a patient with significant residual heart disease and documented recurrent attacks of RF. Consequently, the duration of secondary prophylaxis must be adapted to each patient, depending on the risk of RF recurrence. Several factors can influence the risk of RF recurrence, including:

— the age of the patient
— the presence of RHD
— the time elapsed from the last attack
— the number of previous attacks
— the degree of crowding in the family
— a family history of RF/RHD
— the socioeconomic and educational status of the individual
— the risk of streptococcal infection in the area
— whether a patient is willing to receive injections
— the occupation and place of employment of the patient (school teachers, physicians, employees in crowded areas).

Such decisions can be facilitated using the general recommendations in Table 11.2.

Special situations

Penicillin prophylaxis for recurrent attacks of RF should be continued during pregnancy. There is no evidence of teratogenicity associated

Table 11.2
Suggested duration of secondary prophylaxis*

Category of patient	Duration of prophylaxis
Patient without proven carditis.	For 5 years after the last attack, or until 18 years of age (whichever is longer).
Patient with carditis (mild mitral regurgitation or healed carditis).	For 10 years after the last attack, or at least until 25 years of age (whichever is longer).
More severe valvular disease.	Lifelong.
After valve surgery.	Lifelong.

* See Text. These are only recommendations and must be modified by individual circumstances as warranted

with benzathine benzylpenicillin. The sulfa drugs are *not* recommended because of the potential risk to the fetus. The teenage years present a special problem with adherence to any prophylactic regime; special efforts should be made at this crucial period when the risk of recurrence remains relatively high. Special regimens for patients with RHD must be used for bacterial endocarditis prophylaxis, as secondary RF prevention regimens are not appropriate for preventing endocarditis (see Chapter 12, *Infective endocarditis*). Finally, it should be remembered that even though patients have a prosthetic heart valve they remain susceptible to recurrences of rheumatic fever, but caution must be taken in recommending intramuscular benzathine penicillin G for patients with a prosthetic valve receiving warfarin or another form of anticoagulant.

Penicillin allergy and penicillin skin testing

The incidences of allergic and anaphylactic reactions to monthly benzathine penicillin injections are 3.2% and 0.2% respectively; fatal reactions are rare (*9, 10*). The risk of a serious reaction is reduced in children under the age of 12 years, and the duration of prophylaxis does not appear to increase the risk of an allergic reaction (*1–3*). The long-term benefits of benzathine penicillin therapy in preventing RF far outweigh the risk of a serious allergic reaction (*1–5*).

The overall incidence of hypersensitivity reactions has been estimated to be 2–5% (*10*). The most common allergic reactions are manifest as skin rashes. Anaphylaxis is rare and occurs in only about 0.2% of cases (*11*). It should be emphasized that what appear to be clinical "anaphylactic reactions" have been reported most often in patients with severe RHD. Because of poor cardiac function these patients are more susceptible to vaso-vagal reactions and are at high risk of life-threatening arrhythmias (*9*). Resuscitation can be difficult. Yet such instances do not represent true anaphylaxis. While true anaphylactic reactions can occur in individuals without RHD, the risk is low (*9*, *10*). It has been suggested that the risk of true anaphylaxis is less than the risk of recurrence of RF in some populations (*9*).

Penicillin skin testing is an acceptable and usually accurate method to determine whether a person is at risk of having an immediate reaction to penicillin (*10*, *12*, *13*). Only 10–20% of patients reporting penicillin allergy are truly allergic when assessed by skin testing (*10*, *12*, *14*). Acute allergic reactions are rare in patients with negative skin tests and virtually all patients with a negative skin test can receive penicillin prophylaxis without serious sequelae (*10–13*). However, penicillin skin testing also has an adverse reaction rate of 0.3–1.2%. It is generally considered safe when performed properly, although rare instances of anaphylactic shock have been reported (*14*, *15*).

Health-care providers should take a careful history regarding previous allergic reaction, not only to benzathine penicillin, but also to other beta-lactam antibiotics (such as ampicillin, amoxicillin, cephalosporins, etc.). If a patient has a convincing history of a severe immediate allergic reaction to penicillin (oral or intramuscular), skin testing is *not* advocated and a non-beta-lactam antimicrobial should be used (e.g. erythromycin, sulfa drugs) (*5*, *10*, *12*).

An emergency kit for treating anaphylaxis should be available in any clinical setting where intramuscular penicillin is administered. Although a positive history of penicillin allergy may not always be reliable, it is nevertheless recommended that all patients who are to receive secondary prophylaxis are carefully questioned as to whether they are allergic to penicillin. All health workers dispensing secondary prophylaxis should also be trained in performing the penicillin skin test (*15–17*) and in treating anaphylaxis. If a hypersensitivity reaction of any degree develops during prophylaxis a different antibiotic should be used in the future.

References

1. Lue HC et al. Rheumatic fever recurrences: controlled study of 3-week versus 4-week benzathine penicillin prevention programs. *Journal of Pediatrics*, 1986, **108**:299–304.

2. Dajani AS. Adherence to physicians' instructions as a factor in managing streptococcal pharyngitis. *Pediatrics*, 1996, **97**(6 Pt 2):976–980.

3. Wood HF et al. Rheumatic fever in children and adolescents. A long term epidemiological study of subsequent prophylaxis, streptococcal infections, and clinical sequelae. III. Comparative effectiveness of three prophylaxis regimens in preventing streptococcal infections and rheumatic recurrences. *Annals of Internal Medicine*, 1964, **60**(2) Suppl 5:31–46.

4. American Heart Association. Treatment of acute streptococcal pharyngitis and prevention of rheumatic fever: a statement for health professionals. *Pediatrics*, 1995, **96**(4 Pt 1):758–764.

5. *WHO model prescribing information. Drugs used in the treatment of streptococcal pharyngitis and prevention of rheumatic fever.* Geneva, World Health Organization, 1999 (WHO/EDM/PAR/99.1).

6. Stollerman GH, Russoff JH, Hirschfield I. Prophylaxis against group A streptococci in rheumatic fever. The use of single monthly injection of benzathine penicillin G. *New England Journal of Medicine*, 1955, **252**:787–792.

7. Bass JW et al. Serum levels of penicillin in basic trainees in the US Army who received intramuscular penicillin G benzathine. *Clinical Infectious Diseases*, 1996, **22**(4):727–728.

8. Kaplan EL et al. Pharmacokinetics of benzathine penicillin G: serum levels during the 28 days after intramuscular injection of 1 200 000 units. *Journal of Pediatrics*, 1989, **115**:146–150.

9. International Rheumatic Fever Study Group. Allergic reactions to long-term benzathine penicillin prophylaxis for rheumatic fever. *Lancet*, 1991, **337**:1308–1310.

10. Markowitz M, Lue HC. Allergic reactions in rheumatic fever patients on long-term benzathine penicillin G: the role of skin testing for penicillin allergy. *Pediatrics*, 1996, **97**(S):981–983.

11. Idsoe O et al. Nature and extent of penicillin reactions, with particular reference to fatalities from anaphylactic shock. *Bulletin of the World Health Organization*, 1968, **38**:159–188.

12. Salkind AR et al. Is this patient allergic to penicillin? An evidence-based analysis of the likelihood of penicillin allergy. *Journal of the American Medical Association*, 2001, **285**(19):2498–2505.

13. Redelmeier DA, Sox HC. The role of skin testing for penicillin allergy. *Archives of Internal Medicine*, 1990, **150**(9):1939–1945.

14. Warrington RJ et al. The value of skin testing for penicillin allergy in inpatient population: analisis of the subsequent patient management. *Allergy Asthma Procedings*, 2000, **21**(5):297–299.

15. Forrest DM et al. Introduction of a practice guidelines for penicillin skin testing improves the appropriateness of antibiotic therapy. *Clinical Infectious Diseases*, 2001, **32**(12):1685–1690.

16. Adkinson NF. Tests for immunological drug reactions. In: Rose NR, Friedman H, eds. *Manual of clinical immunology.* Washington, DC, American Society of Microbiology, 1980:822–832.

17. Ressler C, Mendelson L. Skin test for diagnosis of penicillin allergy: current status. *Annals of Allergy*, 1987, **59**:167–170.

12. Infective endocarditis

Introduction

Infective endocarditis poses a special threat for individuals with chronic rheumatic valvular disease, or who have had prosthetic valves implanted because of rheumatic heart disease (RHD). Superimposed upon chronic RHD, infective endocarditis can significantly increase the morbidity and mortality rates in either of these categories of patients. For these patients, prophylaxis for the infective endocarditis is thus recommended. However, individuals who have had rheumatic fever (RF), but who have no evidence of damage to heart valves, do *not* require endocarditis prophylaxis (*1–4*).

Infective endocarditis rarely occurs *without* underlying cardiac pathology, either congenital or acquired. An example of an acquired pathology is seen in intravenous drug users. Even though these individuals usually have normal valvular anatomy, infective endocarditis is not uncommon in this group, particularly of the tricuspid valve. Patients with congenital heart disease also have a higher risk of developing endocarditis. Although a discussion of the risks of infective endocarditis in individuals with congenital heart disease is beyond the scope of this discussion, one principle is that fluid turbulence results in endothelial damage, whether the congenital lesion is valvular, as in congenital bicuspid aortic valves, or a ventricular septal defect. In patients with rheumatic valvular heart disease, infective endocarditis usually occurs in the mitral or aortic valves since these are the most commonly damaged heart valves.

Pathogenesis of infective endocarditis[1]

For the vast majority of patients who develop infective endocarditis (either with bacteria or with fungi), normal laminar blood flow is converted into turbulent flow across the defect. This occurs in patients with rheumatic valvular damage, for example. Although the right-side heart valve is less commonly involved, right-side endocarditis could pose a threat to a patient with either tricuspid or pulmonary valve damage that resulted from RF.

Studies with animal models suggest that turbulent flow may lead to injury and/or disruption of the vascular endothelium or endocardium. As a consequence, a matrix of platelets and fibrin is laid down to form a sterile vegetation. If significant bacteremia then occurs, and bacteremia is common in humans, circulating microorganisms become

---

[1] Source: (*3*).

enmeshed in the initially sterile vegetation and form a nidus of infection. One of the most important factors determining whether bacteria infect sterile vegetation may be the concentration of bacteria circulating through the bloodstream during bacteremia. Early studies also suggested that Gram-positive oral flora, such as viridans group streptococci, had a greater affinity for the vascular endothelium and endocardium than did Gram-negative organisms. This correlated well with clinical observations that Gram-negative organisms frequently cause urinary tract infections, yet rarely cause infective endocarditis. However, investigators caution that understanding of the infective process is incomplete, and point to studies demonstrating that details of the intercellular interactions are species-dependent.

Microbial agents causing infective endocarditis[1]

In the first half of the twentieth century, the most common organisms recovered from individuals with documented infective endocarditis were the alpha-hemolytic streptococci normally found in the oral cavity and upper respiratory tract. This pattern changed in the latter half of that century, with an increase in the number of episodes of infective endocarditis associated with staphylococci, particularly in industrialized countries. Increasingly, *Staphylococcus aureus* and coagulase-negative staphylococci were recovered from infective endocarditis patients, probably because the patients had undergone medical or surgical procedures that required extended hospitalizations. In immunocompromised patients, whether from tumor chemotherapy or from acquired conditions like HIV/AIDS, infective endocarditis has also been associated with other unusual organisms. In most published studies, staphylococci and viridans streptococci were found in more than 50% of the cases, but other organisms are being recovered from patients more frequently, including group D enterococci, gram-negative organisms, and the HACEK organisms (*Haemophilus*, *Actinobacillus*, *Cardiobacterium*, *Eikenella*, and *Kingella*). Similarly, yeast and fungi are also more common for reasons previously mentioned. In developing countries, the continuing predominance of viridans streptococci in patients with endocarditis has been attributed to the poor dental hygiene among children and adults in socially and economically disadvantaged populations.

Clinical and laboratory diagnosis of infective endocarditis[1]

Even in industrialized countries, it has been estimated that a primary-care physician may see only one patient with endocarditis during his/

---

[1] Sources: (*1–7*).

her career. Since the clinical signs and symptoms commonly associated with infective endocarditis are often nonspecific and overlap with many other illnesses, a diagnosis of infective endocarditis can be difficult using clinical observations alone. In 1994, to facilitate patient evaluation, more objective clinical criteria were published for assessing infective endocarditis (6). It is beyond the scope of this document to discuss the use of these criteria in detail. However, as with the Jones Criteria for RF, using clinical criteria to diagnose infective endocarditis is fraught with pitfalls.

It thus important to confirm clinical suspicions of endocarditis with data from the microbiology laboratory. If there are no supporting microbiology laboratory facilities, or if existing ones are substandard, this makes a diagnosis of endocarditis especially difficult. A complicating factor is that patients with nonspecific symptoms at the onset of infective endocarditis are often given antibiotics or take antibiotics on their own. Consequently, even with microbiology laboratory facilities, it can be difficult to confirm a suspected infection. Laboratory studies for assisting the clinician can be divided into two major categories. First, the blood culture is a *sine qua non* for confirming a diagnosis of infective endocarditis. Since the bacteremia associated with endocarditis is thought to be qualitatively continuous, there is no need for the clinician to wait for temperature elevations to obtain blood cultures. It is important to obtain more than a single blood culture (it has been proposed that three samples are sufficient) *before* any antibiotic therapy is initiated. The volume of blood taken for laboratory culture evaluation can be important even in children.

It is more difficult for the clinician to manage a patient with infective endocarditis if the underlying organism has not been identified. This is a problem in locations where there are no fully operational microbiology laboratories. There is a consensus that, at least in local or regional referral hospitals, it is important that the laboratories be equipped for this important task. Other laboratory tests, such as measuring the erythrocyte sedimentation rate or levels of C-reactive protein or other acute-phase reactants, are often helpful for following the clinical course of patients, but are nonspecific measures of inflammation and are not pathognomonic of infective endocarditis. The same is true for the white blood count and differential. Haematuria, casts (or other signs of nephritis) and even small numbers of bacteria (especially staphylococci) in the urine are also helpful adjuncts in making a diagnosis of infective endocarditis.

The technique of echocardiography is potentially the most useful "laboratory" examination in the diagnosis and management of individuals with infective endocarditis. In adults, the resolution and sensitivity of echocardiography can be considerably improved by employing transoesophageal echocardiography. In children, or very thin adults, transthoracic echocardiography may suffice. It is beyond the scope of this document to completely discuss the advantages and disadvantages of this important diagnostic tool. While the identification of a vegetation can be most helpful in establishing the diagnosis, the failure to demonstrate the vegetation by echocardiography does not eliminate the disease from consideration.

It is not uncommon for individuals with endocarditis to present with embolic phenomena. There may be either massive emboli or small emboli producing vague and nonspecific complaints over a period of time. Therefore, the clinician must investigate other organ systems for evidence of embolic phenomena.

Medical and surgical management of infective endocarditis[1]

The most important aspects of the medical management of patients with infective endocarditis are a correct diagnosis and the eradication of the causative microorganism. For these reasons, a positive blood culture remains the "gold standard" for assisting clinicians to plan antibiotic therapy. Although it is possible to make an "educated guess" about the identity of the causative organism, the antibiotic sensitivities of these organisms can vary, not only between countries and cities, but even between hospitals within the same city. Consequently, the antibiotic susceptibility of a causative organism should be tested in a laboratory. Although such laboratories may not always be present in local clinics, a regional referral hospital should be able to perform the tests. Such tests are important to the outcome and can indirectly reduce morbidity and mortality. The importance of performing antibiotic susceptibility tests is underscored by the continuing increase in antibiotic resistance among even the most commonly isolated pathogens associated with infectious endocarditis (e.g. methicillin resistant *Staphylococcus aureus* (MRSA) and vancomycin resistant enterococci (VRE)).

The medical treatment of endocarditis with antibiotics depends upon the microorganism, its sensitivity, and the extent of the involvement. For example, individuals who have myocardial abscess formation will require different considerations than those who have only valvular involvement. The duration of therapy must be sufficiently long to ensure the bacterial infection is cured. Many national cardiac societies

---

[1] Sources: (*2, 3, 6*).

have published recommendations for therapy of infective endocarditis and duration of the treatment. Treatment is essentially always parenteral; oral therapy is less desirable because of the potential for suboptimal patient compliance and the distinct possibility of irregular absorption from the gastrointestinal tract. In addition to antimicrobial therapy, supportive care for complications such as heart failure is important.

If medical management is not effective, surgery must be considered whenever possible. Assuming surgical facilities are accessible, there are several indications for considering prompt surgical intervention, including:

— the persistence of bacteremia by blood culture after four or five days of what should be adequate antibiotic therapy;
— the occurrence of major or multiple continuing embolic phenomena;
— in individuals with valvular heart disease, the presence of significantly increasing valvular dysfunction (i.e. more regurgitation), leading to heart failure.

In individuals with prosthetic valve endocarditis, the criteria are considerably different as this situation is more difficult to treat with antibiotics alone, particularly if there is an annular abscess, for example. The need for surgery is more obvious in these situations. Generally speaking, surgery is not contra-indicated in active infection, and may be the sole life-saving procedure available.

Prophylaxis for the prevention of infective endocarditis in patients with rheumatic valvular heart disease[1]

No controlled study has adequately demonstrated that antibiotic prophylaxis prior to dental or surgical procedures is efficacious in preventing endocarditis. However, numerous reports do confirm that antibiotic prophylaxis reduces the occurrence of bacteremia. Since bacteremia necessarily precedes actual endocarditis, it has been assumed that reducing the occurrence of bacteremia reduces the risk of developing infective endocarditis. Accordingly, while specifics may differ, prophylaxis for infective endocarditis is widely recommended by national cardiac societies around the world.

Prophylaxis for preventing endocarditis has become less complicated. Fifty years ago, three or four days of antibiotic prophylaxis was recommended in advance of a dental or surgical procedure, whereas

---

[1] Sources: (1–5).

Table 12.1

Dental procedures for which endocarditis prophylaxis is recommended[a]

— dental extractions
— periodontal procedures (e.g. surgery, scaling, etc.)
— dental implant placement or replacement
— gingival surgery
— initial placement of orthodontic appliances, but *not* routine adjustments
— dental cleaning when gingival bleeding is expected
— endodontic instrumentation
— intraligamentary local anesthetic injections.

[a] Source: (*1*).

Table 12.2

Dental procedures for which endocarditis prophylaxis is not recommended[a]

— "restorative" dentistry (filling cavities)
— procedures associated with shedding primary teeth
— adjusting orthodontic appliances
— taking oral radiographs
— removing post-operative sutures.

[a] Source: (*1*).

Table 12.3

Other procedures for which endocarditis prophylaxis is recommended[a]

— surgical procedures that involve respiratory tract mucosa (e.g. tonsillectomy)
— bronchoscopy with a rigid bronchoscope
— sclerotherapy for esophageal varices
— oesophageal stricture dilatation
— surgical procedures on intestinal mucosa or biliary tract
— prostate surgery
— cystoscopy and urethral dilation.

[a] Source: (*1*).

current recommendations are for only one or two doses prior to the procedure. It should recognized that individuals who have had RF, but have no evidence of valvular heart disease, do *not* require prophylaxis to prevent infective endocarditis. On the other hand, individuals with rheumatic valvular disease should be given prophylaxis for dental procedures and for surgery of infected or contaminated tissues. Several studies have shown that the use of oral antiseptic solutions (e.g. phenolated oral mouth wash, Betadine mouth wash) can reduce oral flora and reduce bacteremia following dental extraction. While this can be used as an adjunct just prior to dental procedures, it should never replace the use of antibiotics for appropriate indications for prevention.

Table 12.4
Other procedures for which endocarditis prophylaxis is not routinely needed[a]

— endotracheal intubation
— bronchoscopy with flexible bronchoscope
— tympanostomy tube insertion
— trans-oesophageal echocardiography
— vaginal delivery or hysterectomy
— caesarian-section delivery
— if not infected: urethral catheterization, uterine dilatation and curettage, therapeutic abortion, sterilization procedures, insertion or removal of intrauterine devices
— cardiac catheterization or angioplasty
— circumcision
— biopsy of surgically scrubbed skin.

[a] Source: (1).

Table 12.5
Suggested prophylactic antibiotic regimens for dental, oral, respiratory tract and oesophageal procedures[a]

Situation	Antibiotic	Dose[b]
Standard oral	Amoxicillin	One dose
Parenteral	Ampicillin	One dose (IM or IV)
Penicillin allergy	Clindamycin	One dose
Oral	Cephalexin/Cefadroxil	One dose
Parenteral	Cefazolin	One dose

[a] Modified from sources: (1, 2).
[b] Childrens' doses should never exceed the adult doses.

Table 12.6
Suggested antibiotic prophylaxis regimens for gastrointestinal and genitourinary tract procedures[a]

Situation	Antibiotic	Dose[b]
High risk	Ampicillin plus gentamicin	2 doses
High risk/allergy to penicillin	Vancomycin plus gentamicin	1 dose
Moderate risk	Amoxicillin *or* ampicillin	1 dose
Moderate risk/allergy to penicillin	Vancomycin alone	1 dose

[a] Modified from sources: (1, 2).
[b] Childrens' doses should never exceed the adult dose.

A list of dental and other procedures for which endocarditis prophylaxis is, or is not, recommended is given in Tables 12.1–12.4. Commonly proposed antibiotic prophylaxis regimens are given in Tables 12.5 and 12.6. As shown in Table 12.7, individuals already receiving secondary RF prophylaxis with oral penicillin should *not* be given penicillin for their dental or upper respiratory tract procedures. This

Table 12.7

Comparison of antibiotic prophylaxis for rheumatic fever and bacterial endocarditis

Prophylaxis	*Primary* rheumatic fever	*Secondary* rheumatic fever	Bacterial endocarditis
Purpose	To treat group A streptococcal upper respiratory tract infections and eradicate the organism, to prevent an initial attack of acute RF.	To prevent colonization and/or infection in patients who have had a previous attack of RF; prevents a recurrence of RF.	To prevent or minimize bacteremia in patients with heart disease, to prevent the development of infective endocarditis.
When given?	Intermittently: only when there is group A streptococcal infection.	Continuously: duration varies with individual circumstances (age, sequelae, etc.).	Intermittently: shortly before dental or surgical procedures that could result in bacteremia.
Antibiotics commonly used	Penicillin (oral or intramuscular benzathine). Erythromycin for those allergic to penicillin. *Not sulfa drugs and not tetracycline.*	Oral penicillin twice daily, or intramuscular benzathine penicillin G once every 3–4 weeks. May also use oral sulfadiazine or oral erythromycin if the patient is allergic to penicillin.	Those antibiotics directed toward organisms likely to enter the bloodstream from the surgical or dental site; also dependent on the susceptibilities of bacteria to antibiotics in the local area.

is because of the likely presence of penicillin-resistant microorganisms, particularly in the upper respiratory tract and oral cavity of patients receiving oral penicillin. The development of resistance is less likely in individuals receiving intramuscular benzathine penicillin G for secondary RF prophylaxis. However, some authorities believe that a change to a macrolide or clindamycin is more effective for endocarditis prophylaxis.

Summary

Infective endocarditis remains a significant cause (many times unsuspected) of cardiovascular morbidity and mortality. Although there are no data from controlled studies to support the use of antibiotic prophylaxis to prevent infective endocarditis, it remains the accepted medical/dental standard of care. Clearly, antibiotics have been shown to be able to prevent bacteraemia following dental extraction. Furthermore, proper laboratory facilities and clinical acumen are required to reduce the occurrence of this complication of rheumatic heart disease.

References

1. American Heart Association Committee on the Prevention of Rheumatic Fever, Endocarditis and Kawasaki Disease. Prevention of bacterial endocarditis. *Journal of the American Medical Association*, 1997, **277**:1794–1801.

2. European Society of Cardiology Task Force on Infective Endocarditis. Recommendations for prevention, diagnosis and treatment of infective endocarditis. *Unpublished observations.*

3. **Weinstein L, Brusch JL.** *Infective endocarditis.* New York, USA and Oxford, UK, Oxford University Press, 1996.

4. *Rheumatic fever and rheumatic heart disease. Report of a WHO Study Group.* Geneva, World Health Organization, 1988 (WHO Technical Report Series, No. 764).

5. **Durack DT.** Prevention of infective endocarditis. *New England Journal of Medicine*, 1995, **332**:38–44.

6. **Baltimore RS.** Infective endocarditis in children. *Pediatric Infectious Disease Journal*, 1992, **11**:907–912.

7. **Durack DT, Lukes AS, Bright DK.** New criteria for diagnosis of infective endocarditis: utilization of specific echocardiographic findings. Duke Endocarditis Service. *American Journal of Medicine*, 1994, **96**:200–209.

13. Prospects for a streptococcal vaccine

Early attempts at human immunization

Attempts to prevent group A streptococcal infections by immunization date back to the early years of the twentieth century (*1–4*). However, the vaccines did not appear to prevent primary or recurrent attacks of rheumatic fever (RF), despite the injection of large amounts of crude streptococcal toxins and killed organisms into thousands of subjects. Efforts to develop a vaccine against group A streptococci were placed on a firmer scientific footing with the recognition that the principal virulence factor of group A streptococci was M-protein, a streptococcal wall constituent (*5*), and that opsonic antibodies to M-protein protected animals from lethal challenge. Such antibodies persisted for many years in humans (*6*) and appeared to be the basis of acquired type-specific immunity (*7*). Nevertheless, attempts to develop a safe and effective M-protein vaccine encountered considerable difficulties because of the multiplicity of M-protein serotypes (and genotypes), the toxicity of early M-protein preparations, and the immunological cross-reactivity between M-protein and human tissues, including heart tissue (*8*) and synovium (*9*). Cross-reactivity with synovial tissue is of particular concern, because antigenic "mimicry" is thought to play a central role in the pathogenesis of RF (*10*).

M-protein vaccines in the era of molecular biology

Although our knowledge of the structure and function of M-protein has advanced considerably in recent years (*11–15*), M-protein preparations used in vaccines are still not free of epitopes that elicit immunological cross-reactivity with other human tissues. Antibodies against M-proteins, for example, cross-react with alpha-helical human proteins, such as tropomyosin, myosin and vimentin. Primary structure data have revealed that M-proteins of rheumatogenic streptococcal serotypes, such as serotypes 5, 6, 18 and 19, share similar sequences within their B-repeats, and it is likely that such sequences are responsible for eliciting antibodies that cross-react with epitopes in the heart, brain and joints (*16*). Most of the cross-reactive M-protein epitopes appear to be located in the B-repeats, the A-B flanking regions, or the B-C flanking regions, all of which are some distance from the type-specific N-terminal epitopes (*16–18*).

In contrast, antibodies raised against synthetic N-terminal peptides that correspond to the hypervariable portions of M-protein serotypes 5, 6 and 24 are opsonic, but do not cross-react with human tissue (*17–19*). Further studies have shown that peptide fragments of M-proteins, incorporated into multivalent constructs as hybrid proteins or as individual peptides linked in tandem to unrelated carrier proteins, elicited opsonic and mouse-protective antibodies against multiple serotypes, but did not evoke heart-reactive antibodies (20, 21). Phase I human trials with such vaccines are now in progress.

Since a limited number of streptococcal strains (serotypes) are responsible for most human disease, it has been estimated that a serotype-specific octavalent vaccine would prevent 77% of infections causing RF, 52% of those causing severe infections, and 40% of uncomplicated infections (16). These estimates were based on serotype distribution data from economically developed western countries, and such a vaccine might need to be reconstituted, based on prevalent local strains. Current studies are directed toward utilizing commensal gram-positive bacteria as vaccine vectors (22–23).

Immunization approaches not based on streptococcal M-protein

Targets other than streptococcal M-protein have been proposed as a basis for immunization against RF. One of these is C5a peptidase, an enzyme that cleaves the human chemotactic factor, C5a, and thus interferes with the influx of polymorphonuclear neutrophils at the sites of inflammation (24). Intranasal immunization of mice with a defective form of the streptococcal C5a peptidase reduced the colonizing potential of several different streptococcal M-serotypes (25). A second potential vaccine target is streptococcal pyrogenic exotoxin B (SpeB), a cysteine protease that is present in virtually all group A streptococci. Mice passively or actively immunized with the cysteine protease lived longer than non-immunized animals after infection with group A streptococci (26).

Epidemiological considerations

Once a safe and effective streptococcal vaccine is available many practical issues would need to be addressed. With few exceptions, the highest rates of RF tend to occur in areas with limited resources and public health infrastructure, and ways of delivering a vaccine under such conditions need to be examined. Other issues, such as cost, route of administration, number and frequency of required doses, potential side-effects, stability of the material under field conditions, and durability of immunity, would all influence the usefulness of any vaccine. A mucosal vaccine would obviously be preferable to one requiring injections, and it is likely that multivalent vaccines would need to be reformulated to account for the epidemiology of the local streptococcal strains associated with RF (27, 28). These and other questions await the advent of effective vaccines.

Should current efforts to develop a safe and effective group A streptococcus vaccine succeed, the rational application of the vaccine will require knowledge of the clinical, epidemiological and microbiological characteristics of streptococcal disease in many areas of the world. Continued research into these issues should be given a high priority.

Conclusion

The persistence of RF in many developing countries of the world, the apparent increase in life-threatening invasive group A streptococcus infections in North America and Europe, and the revolution in molecular biology have all spurred attempts to achieve a safe and effective vaccine against group A streptococci. The most promising approaches are M-protein-based, including those using multivalent type-specific vaccines, and those directed at non-type-specific, highly conserved portions of the molecule. Success in developing vaccines may be achieved in the next 5–10 years, but this success would have to contend with important questions about the safest, most economical and most efficacious way in which to employ them, as well as their cost-effectiveness in a variety of epidemilogic and socio-economic conditions.

References

1. Rantz LA, Randall E, Rantz HH. Immunization of human beings with group A hemolytic streptococci. *The American Journal of Medicine*, 1949, 6:424–432.

2. Gill FA. A review of past attempts and present concepts of producing streptococcal immunity in humans. *Quarterly Bulletin of Northwestern Medical School*, 1960, 34:326–339.

3. Wasson VP, Brown EE. Immunization against rheumatic fever. *Journal of Pediatrics*, 1943, 23:24–30.

4. Wilson MG, Swift HF. Intravenous vaccination with hemolytic streptococci: its influence on the incidence of rheumatic fever in children. *American Journal of Diseases of Children*, 1931, 42:42–51.

5. Lancefield RC. Current knowledge of type-specific M antigens of group A streptococci. *Journal of Immunology*, 1962, 89:307–313.

6. Lancefield RC. Persistence of type-specific antibodies in man following infection with group A streptococci. *Journal of Experimental Medicine*, 1959, 110:271–292.

7. Wannamaker LW et al. Studies on immunity to streptococcal infections in Man. *American Journal of Diseases of Children*, 1953, 86:347–348.

8. Dale JB, Beachey EH. Multiple, heart-cross-reactive epitopes of streptococcal M proteins. *Journal of Experimental Medicine*, 1985, 161:113–122.

9. **Baird RW et al.** Epitopes of group A streptococcal M protein shared with antigens of articular cartilage and synovium. *Journal of Immunology*, 1991, **146**:3132–3137.

10. **Zabriskie JB.** Rheumatic fever: a model for the pathological consequences of microbial-host mimicry. *Clinical and Experimental Rheumatology*, 1986, **4**:65–73.

11. **Phillips GN Jr. et al.** Streptococcal M protein: alpha-helical coiled-coil structure and arrangement on the cell surface. *Proceedings of the National Academy of Sciences (USA)*, 1981, **78**:4689–4693.

12. **Fischetti VA et al.** Streptococcal M protein: an antiphagocytic molecule assembled on the cell wall. *Journal of Infectious Diseases*, 1977, **136**(Suppl):S222–S233.

13. **Bisno AL.** Alternate complement pathway activation by group A streptococci: role of M-protein. *Infection and Immunity*, 1979, **26**:1172–1176.

14. **Campo RE, Schultz DR, Bisno AL.** M-proteins of group G streptococci: mechanisms of resistance to phagocytosis. *Journal of Infectious Diseases*, 1995, **171**(3):601–606.

15. **Peterson PK et al.** Inhibition of alternative complement pathway opsonization by group A streptococcal M protein. *Journal of Infectious Diseases*, 1979, **139**:575–585.

16. **Dale JB.** Multivalent group A streptococcal vaccines. In: Stevens DL, Kaplan EL, eds. *Streptococcal infections: clinical aspects, microbiology, and molecular pathogenesis*. New York, Oxford University Press, 2000:390–401.

17. **Dale JB, Seyer JM, Beachey EH.** Type-specific immunogenicity of a chemically synthesized peptide fragment of type 5 streptococcal M protein. *Journal of Experimental Medicine*, 1983, **158**:1727–1732.

18. **Beachey EH, Seyer JM.** Protective and nonprotective epitopes of chemically synthesized peptides of the NH_2-terminal region of type 6 streptococcal M protein. *Journal of Immunology*, 1986, **136**:2287–2292.

19. **Beachey EH et al.** Protective and autoimmune epitopes of streptococcal N protein. *Vaccine*, 1988, **6**(2):192–196.

20. **Dale JB.** Multivalent group A streptococcal vaccine designed to optimize the immunogenicity of six tandem M protein fragments. *Vaccine*, 1999, **17**(2):193–200.

21. **Dale JB et al.** Recombinant, octavalent group A streptococcal M protein vaccine. *Vaccine*, 1996, **14**(10):944–948.

22. **Fischetti VA.** Vaccine approaches to protect against group A streptococcal pharyngitis. In: Fischetti VA et al., eds. *Gram-positive pathogens*. Washington, DC, American Society for Microbiology, 2000:96–104.

23. **Fischetti VA, Hodges WM, Hruby DE.** Protection against streptococcal pharyngeal colonization with a vaccinia:M protein recombinant. *Science*, 1989, **244**:1487–1490.

24. **Cleary PP et al.** Streptococcal C5a peptidase is a highly specific endopeptidase. *Infection and Immunity*, 1992, **60**:5219–5223.

25. **Ji Y et al.** Intranasal immunization with C5a peptidase prevents nasopharyngeal colonization of mice by the group A Streptococcus. *Infection and Immunity*, 1997, **65**(6):2080–2087.

26. **Kapur V et al.** Vaccination with streptococcal extracellular cysteine protease (interleukin-1 beta convertase) protects mice against challenge with heterologous group A streptococci. *Microbial Pathogenesis*, 1994, **16**:443–450.

27. **Martin DR et al.** Acute rheumatic fever in Auckland, New Zealand: spectrum of associated group A streptococci different from expected. *The Pediatric Infectious Disease Journal*, 1994, **13**(4):264–269.

28. **Kaplan EL et al.** A comparison of group A streptococcal serotypes isolated from the upper respiratory tract in the USA and Thailand: implications. *Bulletin of the World Health Organization*, 1992, **70**(4):433–437.

14. The socioeconomic burden of rheumatic fever

The socioeconomic burden of rheumatic fever

Although rheumatic fever (RF) and its most important sequel, rheumatic heart disease (RHD), are worldwide problems, they are most prevalent in developing countries. In these countries, RF accounts for up to 60% of all cardiovascular disease in children and young adults, and it has the potential to undermine national productivity, since young adults are the most productive segment of the population in these countries (1, 2). In addition, 67% of school–aged patients drop out of school due to RF, which stifles their ability to realize their full potential (3).

Moreover, the burden of managing RHD puts additional pressure on the economies of these countries, which are often characterized by a low Gross Domestic Product and Gross National Product. In countries of the African region, for example, the direct medical cost of managing one patient with RHD for six years was estimated to be US$ 17 375 in 1987, increasing to US$ 31 661 with surgical procedures (4, 5). And in Nigeria, it was estimated that the cost of treating one patient with RF was equivalent to the cost of preventing 5.4 cases (3). Adding to the burden on health systems of developing countries are the costs of outside referrals that are often required during the course of treatment.

The results of a study of RF and RHD in 100 low-income patients in Sao Paulo, Brazil, underscored the socioeconomic costs of these diseases (6). With a mean follow-up time of 3.9 years (range, 1–10 years), the patients had a total of 1657 medical consultations, 22 hospital admissions and 4 admissions to an intensive care unit. It was also estimated that RF and RHD patients had a 22% failure rate in school. The socioeconomic costs were also borne by the parents of the patients, with 22% exhibiting absenteeism from work, and about 5% losing their jobs. There are also intangible costs associated with RF and RHD, resulting from premature disability and death, as well as from the loss of intellectual opportunities, with its adverse effects on the socioeconomic development of the family and society. In Brazil, the annual cost of RF to society was estimated to be US$ 51 144 347, approximately equivalent to 1.3% of the average family income.

Besides the more immediate costs of RF and RHD documented by such studies, these diseases could also have distal effects. Already, there are inherent inequities in health-care access and delivery for less-advantaged people in developing countries, and the additional burdens that RF and RHD place on the economies of these countries could exacerbate these inequities. Potentially, the most cost-effective strategy for ameliorating the impact of RF and RHD on the economies and health-care systems of developing countries is the secondary prevention of RF.

Cost-effectiveness of control programmes

In low-income and middle-income countries with a high prevalence of RF and RHD, prevention and control programmes must compete for limited resources, and it is therefore crucial that available resources be committed efficiently to guarantee the success and sustainability of such programmes. As a programme design strategy, it is advisable to attempt small-scale pilot programmes before initiating large-scale national control programmes, as the lessons learnt from pilot schemes can, in addition to many other benefits, prevent the waste of scarce resources (2, 7).

The available empirical evidence underscores the intuitive notion that secondary prevention programmes are the most cost-effective, when compared with primary prevention programmes and programmes focusing on managing the cardiovascular complications of RF. For example, the cost of averting one death and gaining 37 DALYs[1] that would have been lost was estimated to be US$ 40920 using primary prophylaxis alone, US$ 12750 using tertiary prevention strategies (including cardiac surgeries), but only US$ 5520 using secondary prophylaxis (8). In New Zealand, the average hospital costs for treating RHD (which included the cost of surgery) accounted for 87% of total expenditures for RF and RHD in 1985, whereas the ambulatory component of care accounted for only 13% of total expenditure share (9). Management of chronic RHD alone can take as much as 71% of the total national allocation for treating RF and RHD (10), and much of this expenditure could be prevented with vigorous efforts at cheaper secondary prevention programmes.

These studies emphasize that national prevention programmes based on secondary prophylaxis have the potential for considerable cost savings, which could be used to improve the spread and gains of a programme. National control programmes should therefore focus on reducing the need for hospitalization, averting the need for surgery, and improving the quality of life (when RF has been established).

---

[1] The disability-adjusted life years (DALYs) lost is the sum of the number of years of life lost due to premature death, plus the number of years lived with disability, adjusted for the severity of disability.

Such programmes, which are integrated within existing primary health-care systems, have the further potential to reduce the cost burden on patients (7).

No control programme would be complete without strategies for treating acute pharyngitis and acute episodes of RF in endemic, and particularly epidemic, situations. Strategies should be tailored towards local circumstances, however. Evidence has been presented from a simulation study suggested that the most cost-effective strategy was to treat all pharyngitis patients with penicillin (particularly those within an at-risk group), without a strict policy of waiting for the disease to be confirmed by bacterial culture (7, 11). However, this approach has not been confirmed and cannot be advocated until more thorough studies are carried out. In hospital settings where facilities are available, the "culture and treat" strategy has been shown to be cost-effective (12).

References

1. Githang'a D. Rheumatic heart disease (editorial comment). *East African Medical Journal*, 1999, **76**(11):599–600.

2. *Joint WHO/ISFC meeting on RF/RHD control with emphasis on primary prevention, Geneva, 7–9 September 1994*. Geneva, World Health Organization, 1994 (document WHO/CVD 94.1).

3. Jaiyesimi F. Chronic rheumatic heart disease in childhood: its cost and economic implications. *Tropical Cardiology*, 1982, **8**(30):55–59.

4. Olubodun JOB. Acute rheumatic fever in Africa. *Africa Health*, 1994, **16**(5):32–33.

5. Ekra A, Bertrand E. Rheumatic heart disease in Africa. *World Health Forum*, 1992, **13**(4):331–333.

6. Terreri MT et al. Resource utilization and cost of rheumatic fever. *Journal of Rheumatology*, 2001, **28**(6):1394–1397.

7. *The WHO Global Programme for the prevention of RF/RHD. Report of a consultation to review progress and develop future activities*. Geneva, World Health Organization, 2000 (document WHO/CVD/00.1).

8. Michaud CJ et al. Rheumatic heart disease. In: Jamison DT et al., eds. *Disease control priorities in developing countries*. New York, Oxford University Press, **1993**:221–232.

9. Neutze JM. Rheumatic fever and rheumatic heart disease in the Western Pacific Region. *New Zealand Medical Journal*, 1988, **101**: 404–406.

10. North DA et al. Analysis of costs of acute rheumatic fever and rheumatic heart disease in Auckland. *New Zealand Medical Journal*, 1993, **106**:400–403.

11. **Tompkins RT, Burnes DC, Cables WC.** Analysis of the cost-effectiveness of pharyngitis management and acute rheumatic fever prevention. *Annals of Internal Medicine*, 1977, **86**(4):481–492.

12. **Tsevatt J, Kotagal UR.** Management of sore throats in children: a cost-effectiveness analysis. *Archives of Pediatric and Adolescent Medicine*, 1999, **153**:681–688.

15. Planning and implementation of national programmes for the prevention and control of rheumatic fever and rheumatic heart disease

The establishment of a national prevention programme is essential in countries where rheumatic fever (RF) and rheumatic heart disease (RHD) remain significant health problems. Both primary and secondary prevention of RF and RHD have been proven to be safe, feasible and effective in both developed and developing countries (1–12). The overall goal of a national programme should be to reduce morbidity, disabilities and mortality from RF and RHD.

At country level, the planning phase of the programme should include an assessment of the prevalence of RF and RHD and a plan of operation with objectives and approaches adapted to local needs and circumstances. It is important to implement such programmes through the existing national infrastructure of the ministry of health and the ministry of education without building a new administrative mechanism. This would minimize additional costs and prevent unsustainable monolithic programmes (2, 3, 6, 11, 12). Based upon previous experience (1, 2, 11, 12), planning and implementation of national programmes should be based on the following principles:

- There should be a strong commitment at policy level, particularly in the ministries of health and education.
- A national advisory committee should be formed, under the auspices of the ministry of health, with broad representation from all stakeholders, including representatives from a wide spectrum of professional organizations (e.g. cardiologists, paediatricians, family physicians, internal medicine specialists, epidemiologists and nurses).
- Programme implementation should be stepwise. For example, start in one or more defined areas to test whether the methods and procedures are appropriate for the local situation (Phase I), and then gradually extend the programme to provincial (Phase II) and national coverage (Phase III).
- The programme should be service-oriented and emphasize active secondary prevention, and be integrated into the existing health-care systems, particularly primary health care.
- Support from the microbiology laboratory should be optimized at peripheral, intermediate and national levels.
- Suspected outbreaks of group A beta-haemolytic streptococcal infection should be controlled and studied.

The main components of a national programme are:

- secondary prevention activities aimed at preventing the recurrence of acute RF and severe RHD;
- primary prevention activities aimed at preventing the first attack of acute RF;
- health education activities;
- training of health-care providers;
- epidemiological surveillance;
- community involvement.

Secondary prevention activities

Secondary prevention is based on case finding, referral, registration, surveillance, follow-up and regular secondary prophylaxis for RF and RHD patients. A central or a local referral or registration centre should be established in participating areas. Once detected, patients with a history of RF or with RHD are referred to the central or local centre for medical care, follow-up and long-term secondary prophylaxis. Attention should be given to patients who have difficulties in adhering to long-term secondary prophylaxis regimes, or who drop out of the prevention regime (i.e. they miss more than two consecutive injections). For more details see Chapter 11, *Secondary prevention of rheumatic fever*.

Primary prevention activities

Primary prevention is based on the early detection, correct diagnosis and appropriate treatment of individual patients with Group A streptococcal pharyngitis. Vertical programmes for the primary prevention of RF and RHD are not cost effective in developing countries. Such programmes need to part of the routine medical care available and should be integrated in to the existing health infrastructure. Health education to the public, teachers and health personnel would enhance the impact of a primary prevention programme. For more details see Chapter 10, *Primary prevention of rheumatic fever*.

Health education activities

Health education activities should address both primary and secondary prevention. The activities may be organized by trained doctors, nurses or teachers and should be directed at the public, teachers and parents of school-age children. Health education activities should focus on the importance of recognizing and reporting sore throats early; on methods that minimize and avoid the spread of infection; on the benefits of treating sore throats properly; and on the importance of complying with prescribed treatment regimes.

Health education campaigns in schools and in the community are effective methods for communicating health messages and for increasing awareness in schoolchildren and parents. Health messages could be transmitted to parents indirectly by targeting schoolchildren. The involvement of the print and electronic media (radio, TV, newsletters, posters) is vital to the success of such programmes. Patient group meetings are also a potent means of transmitting and networking health information. The commitment of the school and school health service (when available) to the health education of children is of tremendous importance when implementing RF/RHD control programmes.

Training health-care providers

Members of the health team at all levels have clearly identified roles and responsibilities in running RF/RHD prevention programmes, and they should receive appropriate training at regular intervals. Training should be given to physicians, as well as to non-physician health-care providers who are involved in primary or secondary prevention activities. Training programmes should stress the importance of early detection, diagnosis and appropriate treatment of streptococcal pharyngitis, as well as the importance of detecting, treating RF/RHD and monitoring compliance to secondary prophylaxis. Training courses should also include procedures for penicillin skin testing and for treating anaphylactic reactions.

Public health nurses are essential for running RF/RHD prevention programmes in developing countries, particularly in planning, coordinating and implementing such programmes where there is a shortage of available doctors.

Epidemiological surveillance

Surveillance of acute RF and RHD, if incorporated in to the national statistical report, would provide useful information on the epidemiological trends of the disease. Regular analysis and evaluation of the RF and RHD registers would also provide useful information on trends and characteristics of the disease in defined locations. Where resources permit, surveys in school-age children may be conducted to determine prevalence of RF/RHD, the seasonal frequency and distribution of streptococcal pharyngitis, and the levels of antistreptolysin-O titres in the school-age population.

Community and school involvement

The success of a prevention programme depends on the cooperation, effectiveness and dedication of health personnel at all levels, as well as of other members of the community (e.g. health administrators, educational administrators, teachers and community leaders). Most importantly, potential patients themselves and their families must be involved in the control strategies adopted by communities.

As schools play a large part in spreading streptococcal infection, they can also play a large role in its control. Where school health services exists, they should be used to identify children with signs suggestive of RF. Screening schoolchildren for RF is worthwhile in areas with a high prevalence of RHD, and such screening may be carried out by community health workers who have been specially trained for the purpose. Teachers and pupils should also be involved in efforts to improve patient adherence to secondary prophylaxis, as well as in follow-up procedures.

A manual with detailed recommendations for preparing a plan of operation for RF and RHD prevention has been published by the WHO/CVD programme (2).

References

1. *Rheumatic fever and rheumatic heart disease. Report of a WHO Study Group.* Geneva, World Health Organization, 1988 (Technical Report Series, No. 764).

2. *The WHO Global Programme for the prevention of RF/RHD. Report of a consultation to review progress and develop future activities.* Geneva, World Health Organization, 2000 (document WHO/CVD/00.1).

3. **Gordis L.** The virtual disappearance of rheumatic fever in the United States: lessons in the rise and fall of disease. *Circulation*, 1985, **72**(6):1155–1162.

4. **Arguedas A, Mohs E.** Prevention of rheumatic fever in Costa Rica. *Journal of Pediatrics*, 1992, **121**(4):569–572.

5. **Flight RJ.** The Northland rheumatic fever register. *New Zealand Medical Journal*, 1984, **97**:671–673.

6. **Bach JF et al.** 10-year educational programme aimed at rheumatic fever in two French Caribbean islands. *Lancet*, 1996, **347**:644–648.

7. **Neilson G et al.** Rheumatic fever and chronic rheumatic heart disease in Yarrabah aboriginal community, North Queensland. Establishment of a prophylactic program. *Medical Journal of Australia*, 1993, **158**:316–318.

8. **Nordet P et al.** Fiebre reumatica in Ciudad de la Habana, 1972–1982. Incidencia y caracteristicas. [Rheumatic fever in Havana, 1972–1982. Incidence and characteristics.] *Revista Cubana de Pediatria, [Cuban Journal of Pediatrics]* 1988, **60**(2):32–51.

9. **Nordet P et al.** Fiebre reumatica in Ciudad de la Habana, 1972–1982. Prevalencia y caracteristicas. [Rheumatic fever in Havana, 1972–1982. Prevalence and characteristics.] *Revista Cubana de Pediatria, [Cuban Journal of Pediatrics]* 1989, **61**(2):228–237.

10. **Majeed HA et al.** The natural history of acute rheumatic fever in Kuwait: a prospective six-year follow-up report. *Journal of Chronic Diseases*, 1986, **39**(5):361–369.

11. **Strasser T et al.** The community control of rheumatic fever and rheumatic heart disease: report of a WHO international cooperative project. *Bulletin of the World Health Organization*, 1981, **59**(2):285–294.

12. WHO programme for the prevention of rheumatic fever/rheumatic heart disease in 16 developing countries: report from Phase I (1986–1990). *Bulletin of the World Health Organization*, 1992, **70**(2):213–218.

16. Conclusions and recommendations

1. Although proven inexpensive cost-effective strategies for the prevention and control of streptococcal infections and their non-suppurative sequelae, acute rheumatic fever and rheumatic heart disease, are available, these diseases remain significant public-health problems in the world today, particularly in developing countries.

2. Available data suggest that the incidence of group A streptococcal pharyngitis and other infections as well as the prevalence of the asymptomatic carrier state have remained unchanged in both developed and developing countries.

3. The largely ineffective control of RF and RHD in developing countries is associated with poverty, and its associated conditions such as substandard nutrition and overcrowding, and inadequate housing. In addition, weak infrastructure and limited resources for health care also contribute to the poor status of control.

4. Although progress has been made in the understanding of possible pathogenic mechanism(s) responsible for the epidemiology and the development of these non-suppurative sequelae of streptococcal infections, the precise pathogenic mechanism(s) are not identified or understood.

5. The diagnostic criteria for RF and RHD have been reviewed and modifications have been recommended based upon new information and upon the need to offer practical guidelines for diagnosis and management for physicians and for public health authorities. These 2002–2003 World Health Organization criteria for the diagnosis of RF and RHD specifically address:
   - *Primary attacks of rheumatic fever*
   - *Recurrent attacks of rheumatic fever in patients without evidence of rheumatic heart disease*
   - *Recurrent attacks of rheumatic fever in patients with pre-existing rheumatic heart disease.*
   - *Rheumatic (Sydenham) chorea*
   - *Insidious onset carditis associated with rheumatic fever*
   - *Chronic rheumatic heart disease*

6. Clinical history and physical examination remain the mainstay for diagnosing RF and rheumatic valvular heart disease particularly in resource-poor settings. Two-dimensional echo-Doppler and colour flow Doppler echocardiography have a role to play in establishing and clinically following rheumatic carditis and rheumatic valvular heart disease.

7. The clinical microbiology laboratory plays an essential role in rheumatic fever control programs, by facilitating the identification of group A streptococcal infections and providing information of streptococcal types causing the disease. National and regional streptococcal reference laboratories are lacking in many parts of the world and attention needs to be given to establish such laboratories and to assure quality control.

8. Patients with rheumatic valvular disease need timely referral for operative intervention when clinical or echocardiographic criteria are met. Management of RHD in pregnancy depends on the type and severity of valvular disease, and regular followed up and evaluation are mandatory for this purpose.

9. Primary prevention of rheumatic fever consists of the effective treatment of group A beta-hemolytic streptococcal pharyngitis, with the goal of preventing the first attack of rheumatic fever. While it is not always feasible to implement broad-based primary prevention programs in most developing countries, a provision for the prompt diagnosis and effective therapy of streptococcal pharyngitis should be integrated into the existing healthcare facilities.

10. Secondary prevention of rheumatic fever is defined as regular administration of antibiotics (usually benzathine penicillin G given intramuscularly) to patients with a previous history of rheumatic fever/rheumatic heart disease in order to prevent group A streptococcal pharyngitis and a recurrence of acute rheumatic fever. Establishment of registries of known patients has proven effective in reducing morbidity and mortality.

11. Infective endocarditis remains a major threat for individuals with chronic rheumatic valvular disease and also for patients with prosthetic valves. Individuals with rheumatic valvular disease should be given prophylaxis for dental procedures and for surgery of infected or contaminated areas.

12. The establishment of a national RF prevention program is essential in countries where RF and RHD remain significant health problems. It is important to include such programs in national health development plans, and to implement them through the existing national infrastructure of ministries of health and of education without requiring a new administrative framework or health care delivery infrastructure.

13. Well planned and encompassing research studies are required to gather epidemiological data on group A streptococcal infections,

RF and RHD. This can result in the targeting of high risk individuals and populations to make more effective use of often limited financial and human resources. Basic research studies are also needed to further elucidate the pathogenesis mechanisms responsible for the development of the disease process and for development of a cost-effective vaccine.